My Senior Dog

A Complete Guide to Caring for Your Old Dog

Hope Chambers

Paperback Print ISBN 979-8-9876848-5-6

Kindle ISBN 979-8-9876848-4-9

Library of Congress Control Number 2023902381

Print edition—First Addition 2023

Table of Contents

In loving memory of Gizmo. You turned my life upside down, and I thank you every day for it.

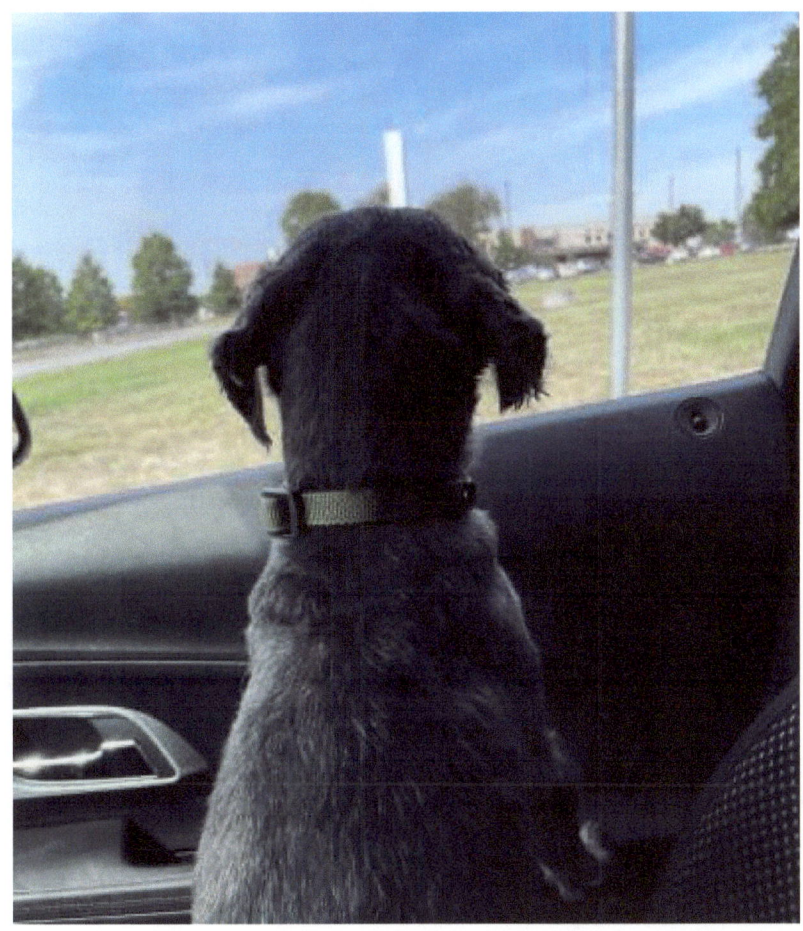

Introduction

Sam seems to be slowing down these days… You wake up in the morning and shuffle down the hallway, eager to greet your best friend. Sam is laying there, staring seamlessly at the wall with milky eyes, he didn't even notice you. As you get closer, he raises his head and wags his tail, but this is not the same ball of energy that used to bound down the hallway to greet you with kisses.

If there is anything that gets him going, it is food! His excited little tail beats against your leg as you prepare his breakfast. He has been losing weight, maybe it is time to give him lunch as well? He starts chomping down immediately, but he seems to struggle when it comes to chewing the bigger pieces.

After breakfast, it is time to potty. It's a beautiful day and a perfect morning for a game of fetch. Sam walks out the door with you but pauses at the stairs. The large grassy backyard has lost its appeal, and he decides that he would rather potty on the deck.

You throw the ball to start a game of fetch, perhaps that will get him moving. He stops and watches the ball bounce, but after a thoughtful moment, he turns around to go back inside. Something just doesn't feel right, but you're going to be late for work. You go to give him a quick kiss on the forehead and realize that he's shivering as he curls up in his bed. It's not that cold, is it? Grabbing a warm blanket, you tuck him in before you leave.

There is no better feeling than arriving home to an ecstatic dog, but today Sam is not waiting, he's asleep again. You wake him up, and he looks at you with all the love in the world. He tries to get up to greet you but quickly loses his balance. Not to worry! You are there to catch him and help him up.

It's time for the routine afternoon walk, an activity that Sam usually loves, but you can tell he is not up for it and the two of you snuggle up in front of the TV instead. Stroking him gently, you notice the tiny gray hairs growing around his muzzle, and you wonder, is Sam really getting old?

These are just a few examples of how your dog may act when they reach their senior years. Most owners are not prepared for these changes, and why should they be? Dogs aren't supposed to get old! The idea that you may have to say goodbye to your dog soon is absolutely terrifying, but it is important that you don't get stuck in this mindset. It may feel as though the end is near, but for your dog, this is just the beginning of their golden year's adventure.

My passion for dog training began when I brought home my first rescued dog. He was the epitome of chaos and my best friend. He changed my life, pushed me out of my comfort zone, and while I healed him, he healed me. He showed me my purpose, and together we set out to learn, train, and help as many people and pups as possible.

The day that I realized he was getting old, I was heartbroken. I immediately hit the books, searching for an immortality potion. Failing that, the least I could do was ensure that I would be able to provide the best care for him. However, even with my new-found knowledge, I still felt so overwhelmed and ill-equipped. Until, as always, he came to my rescue.

I learned to listen and realized that he was showing me exactly what was wrong and what he needed. The last few years we spent together were some of the happiest of my life. The knowledge I gained and the techniques I learned have proved invaluable, and I have been able to use and adapt them to suit the needs of any senior dog.

If you feel that your dog is slowly slipping into their senior years, and you are beginning to lose sleep over it, don't worry! I am here to help you both. This book is packed with all the information and techniques that I have used, adapted, and perfected over the last 30 years. From medical conditions and diet management to grooming tips and dog-approved life hacks, rest assured that you will find your answers here.

Let's dig in!

Chapter 1:

Is My Dog Old?

Believe it or not, the age of your dog is not actually an accurate way to tell whether they are old or not! We have all heard that one dog year is equivalent to seven human years, but this rule doesn't actually translate. Experts have since worked out that the first year of a dog's life is equivalent to fifteen human years. The second year is equivalent to nine human years. From there on, each year can be judged at around five human years.

However, even with this myth busted, there is still no set rule or age that marks your dog old. Just like humans, aging is slow and subtle, and the rate at which individuals age varies greatly. Genetics, trauma, illness, and lifestyle all contribute to the body's general health and the rate at which it declines. Dogs, from the same litter, can even age at a different rate. So, how on earth are you supposed to prepare for your dog's senior years, and how will you know when they get there? Understanding your dog and being aware of the physical and mental changes they may go through is key. Let's take a look at some of the most common signs.

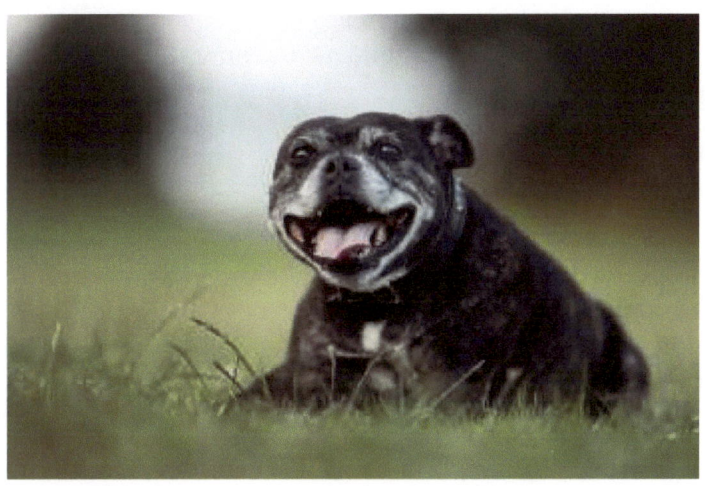

Aging Your Dog

With the exception of large and giant dogs, the general rule of thumb is to assume that your dog will enter their senior years at the age of seven. At this point, veterinary checks should be conducted at least once a year, and lifestyle changes need to be considered.

Size Matters

Yes… size matters. Small dogs generally live longer than their larger counterparts.

Small and toy breeds, under twenty pounds, typically reach their senior years when they are around ten years of age. Medium dog breeds, under fifty pounds, become seniors at seven years of age. Large and giant dog breeds enter their senior years at around five years of age.

Scientists are still unable to provide a concrete reason as to why this happens, but they do have a theory on why large dogs are more susceptible to age-related medical conditions. Their bodies need to grow at a much faster rate, which makes them more likely to experience abnormal cell growth. This cell growth places strain on the internal organs, which can cause early aging and a quicker decline of the immune system.

This is why it is so important to understand your dog's breed!

Effects of Injury and Illness

Injuries and illness can contribute to early aging or at least age-related conditions in pets. Dogs that have suffered injuries, particularly in the legs, are more likely to develop joint stiffness and arthritis at a much younger age. This will cause them to slow down earlier, which makes them prone to conditions such as obesity.

Severe and prolonged illnesses such as diabetes, cancers, and heart conditions put immense strain on the body. They suppress the immune system and can affect the health of internal organs. Making age-related conditions more likely to occur at a younger age.

Effects of Trauma

Mental and emotional trauma can also cause premature aging in dogs. Continuous fear and stress can cause hormonal imbalances, which can lead to a suppressed immune system and impact the heart and other vital organs. The short-term effects of stress, such as weight loss and vomiting, are the most noticeable and will often subside once the dog is in a happier environment.

Unfortunately, the long-term effects only show themselves later in life, and dogs can experience age-related conditions such as heart disease and diabetes before their senior years.

Premature graying in humans is a clear sign of stress, and studies have proved that dogs can experience the same thing! The little gray hairs that naturally form around their muzzles when they age can start to show in chronically stressed dogs as young as four years old.

Behavioral Changes

Behavioral changes in senior dogs are typically passed off as mental decline due to age. However, this is usually not the case. With the exception of cognitive dysfunction syndrome and canine dementia, most of these changes are a direct response to the physical changes they are experiencing.

Disinterest

General disinterest is one of the first behavioral signs owners notice in aging dogs. They will often become reluctant to partake in physically demanding activities such as walks or playing fetch. Their toys may become less exciting and the prospect of jumping up onto the couch to snuggle with you is no longer appealing.

This disinterest is likely due to a physical cause. If your dog is experiencing joint stiffness or arthritis, they will try to avoid going on walks, jumping, and other activities that are likely to cause them pain. Dental conditions, infections, and disturbed sleep cycles can cause disinterest.

How Can I Help?

Try to find out what is causing the disinterest and adjust your routine and lifestyle accordingly. Cut your walks shorter and pick up your dog when they need to jump onto the couch or into the car. Provide them with mentally stimulating toys, and swap out the hard chew toys for soft squeaky ones!

When to Worry

If the changes have not helped, and they become disinterested in more activities, food, and even people, it is time to visit your veterinarian. They may be struggling with a much more serious medical condition.

Disorientation

Disorientation is always worrying. You may notice that your dog is getting "stuck" or lost in areas that they should be familiar with. They will often stare blankly at walls, be unable to recognize familiar people, and have a harder time completing everyday tasks.

Depending on the behaviors they are displaying, this could be due to physical conditions such as a loss of eyesight or hearing. A more concerning cause is cognitive dysfunction syndrome and canine dementia.

How Can I Help?

Take your dog for a check-up to confirm the cause of the disorientation. You can then make the necessary lifestyle changes. Decluttering your home, keeping furniture in the same place, and closing off access to dangerous areas will help your dog to navigate their surroundings safely. Older dogs will struggle to adapt to frequent changes, so it is important to keep up a routine and avoid stressful situations.

When to Worry

If the disorientation gets worse or if you suspect that your dog is going senile, you need to speak to your veterinarian! They will be able to direct you on the next steps, medications, and lifestyle changes that you need to implement. Without proper treatment, your dog is at risk of harming themselves and others.

Aggression and Fear

Aggressive behaviors in senior dogs are linked directly to fear or pain. If your dog has begun to snap at you when you approach them, you may find that they are suffering from hearing or sight loss. They do not know that you are approaching, so they get scared when they suddenly sense you. If they have begun to bite or snap when you touch them, they are likely experiencing pain. This response is especially noticeable if you have other dogs in the household that like to play a little too rough with them.

How Can I Help?

Firstly, find the cause! If they are experiencing sensory decline, announce yourself before you approach them to keep them from getting scared. Provide them with a safe space to retreat to when they begin to feel uncomfortable with their surroundings. Crates, kennels, and even dog beds with sides work wonderfully.

If your pup is experiencing pain from an infection, injury, or underlying condition, your veterinarian will be able to locate the source and treat it accordingly. Be sure to keep younger, boisterous dogs away from your senior dog while they recover.

When to Worry

If there is no underlying physical cause and your dog continues to become more aggressive, it could be a sign of canine dementia. If this is the case, it is important to isolate your senior from other household pets and unfamiliar guests. This is especially vital if you are not there to supervise the interactions. This will reduce the risk of your dog harming others. Dementia is the worst-case scenario, and you will need your veterinarian to assist you with appropriate treatments.

It's important to remember that isolation is not a punishment! You should provide your dog with all the comforts they are used to, including plenty of toys and tons of love. Once you begin to see improvement, you can allow them more freedom to interact with others.

Abnormal Sleeping Patterns

This refers to dogs that have trouble sleeping through the night or tend to sleep for long periods during the day. Some dogs may do both. There are a couple of reasons why this could happen.

Dogs naturally lose their stamina as they age. If your pup sleeps well through the night but takes a few extra naps during the day, then let them sleep! It's completely normal behavior.

A lack of exercise can contribute to a sleepless night. Countless owners quit their regular routines as soon as their dog reaches their senior years. If your dog is sleeping away their boredom during the day, they are likely too energetic to sleep at night.

Dogs that are experiencing discomfort from stiff joints and limbs may struggle to get comfortable. The constant need to toss and turn will disturb their sleep patterns.

How Can I Help?

Heavy dogs should be given thick, comfortable mattresses to sleep on to ensure they are not laying on the hard floor. This will help to alleviate any discomfort they experience from aching joints.

Regular exercise and mentally stimulating tasks are an absolute must. You don't need to run your dog, but short, slow walks can make all the difference.

When to Worry

If your dog is sleeping for hours at a time and is struggling to wake up, it is time to visit your veterinarian. If they start to display symptoms of sleep deprivation such as irritability, disorientation, and forgetfulness, it is time to visit your veterinarian!

Most behavioral changes in senior dogs are subtle and take time to develop. If you catch them early, they can be remedied at home with little effort. However, if you ever feel unsure, it is best to take your dog for a check-up. Any extreme or abrupt behavioral changes should be treated as an emergency.

Physical Changes

As your dog ages, it is only natural for them to experience physical changes. Their bodies begin to take strain, their metabolism slows and their immune system degrades. Most of these changes don't require medical attention, but it is important to monitor them and make the appropriate lifestyle changes to keep them comfortable.

Cold Sensitivity

The ability to regulate body temperature is one of the struggles your aging dog may experience. This is generally age-related, but their weight, general health and fur can all contribute.

A dog's fur is a dog's clothes. Without it, they struggle to keep warm. As they age, their hair follicles age. You may find that their fur begins to thin out, and they develop graying around their muzzles. Muscle mass generates heat and provides insulation, and body fat is used as a backup energy source. Senior dogs that experience weight loss will likely lose muscle as well and without extra fat for energy, they have a harder time staying warm.

How Can I Help?

It's time to buy some sweaters! I like to have a range of sweaters, from thin indoor ones to thick outdoor coats. Booties and socks are a great way to keep your pup's feet and joints warm and are especially important in snowy weather. Warm blankets and heated beds will help them to stay warm throughout the night.

Now that their body doesn't need to work as hard at keeping them warm, it can focus on regulating important bodily functions. You will often notice a quick improvement in their general health.

When to Worry

If you find that your dog is shaking uncontrollably and struggling to get warm even with a sweater on, you should take them for a check-up. This could be due to an underlying medical condition, such as a neurological disease. Hypothermia, bronchitis, and pneumonia can develop if your dog remains cold for long periods of time. These are all dangerous conditions that can become fatal if not treated.

Vision Loss

If you notice that your dog has started to stare blankly at the wall, or doesn't recognize you until you walk closer, then they are likely losing their vision. Vision loss happens gradually, and most owners don't even notice it until their dog starts walking straight into walls! This can be caused by cataracts which reduce vision or by nuclear sclerosis which only affects depth perception. A white, hazy film over the eyes is apparent in both cases.

How Can I Help?

Vision loss can be treatable depending on the cause. If caught early, eye drops and minor surgery can prevent it from progressing further. Cataracts can be surgically removed, but this is not often done with older, high-risk dogs that have other medical conditions.

The best way to combat the effects of vision loss is by making your home blind friendly. Keep large items such as furniture in the same place and remove any clutter that could trip up your dog. Block off any dangerous areas such as pools and stairs to avoid any injuries.

If your pup is really struggling to see, it is time to take advantage of their other senses. You can mark different rooms in your house by putting down different textured mats or using different scents. This will help them to recognize where they are through smell and touch.

When to Worry

If your dog is losing their vision at a rapid rate, or if they are having frequent eye infections, you will need to take them through for a check-up. They could be suffering from diabetes or sudden acquired retinal degeneration syndrome (S.A.R.D.S.). Both of which can have incredibly painful symptoms that need to be treated immediately.

Hearing Loss

Hearing loss is another common symptom of aging that most owners don't notice until it is severe. Your dog may stop obeying your commands, and they will often bark for no reason. You may find that they are easily frightened and will snap at you or other dogs when approached too quickly. It happens gradually and while it is usually an age-related symptom, it can be worsened by ear infections, thick fur around the ears, and underlying medical conditions.

How Can I Help?

A check-up should be done to ensure that they aren't suffering from an ear infection. If this is the case, treatment should help alleviate any pain and can restore some of their hearing.

Deaf dogs can still detect vibration, and you can get their attention by clapping or knocking on a hard surface. However, this doesn't really help if they can't figure out what you are trying to tell them. Training hand signals from an early age can greatly assist in communication.

When to Worry

If you find that your dog is scratching their ears, often leading to wounds or bleeding, they could have a serious inner ear infection. Nerve damage from injuries can also contribute to hearing loss and an annoying pins and needles feeling. This needs to be treated as soon as possible.

Appetite and Weight Changes

As your dog's metabolism slows, you may find that they are losing or gaining weight. This can occur even when they are still eating the same-sized meals with the same calories.

Weight loss is generally due to a reduction in muscle mass or poor absorption of nutrients. A loss of appetite is a common symptom of digestive issues and dental pain. Weight gain is commonly due to a lack of regular exercise. Your dog is no longer expanding the amount of energy that they are getting from their food!

How Can I Help?

A change of diet and exercise routine is the best remedy here. We will work through this in-depth in the following chapters. If you are concerned that your dog may be suffering from a dental condition, it is time to visit your vet!

When to Worry

If your dog loses more than 10% of their body weight, it is time to worry! Internal parasites, organ failure and disease can all contribute to this drastic drop. These are serious conditions that should be treated immediately.

Incontinence

Incontinence is one of the most frustrating physical changes in senior dogs. Your dog may struggle to hold it in for long periods of time and in severe cases, they are unable to hold it in at all. The nerves that control the bladder will deteriorate with age, and the outflow valve is unable to fully close. In this case, you may find small puddles of urine around the house or in your dog's bed.

How Can I Help?

Regular potty breaks and indoor potty areas are usually enough to keep your house clean and your dog happy. In more serious cases, you can use specialized doggy diapers. If your dog is messing on themselves, it is important to keep up with regular baths. Not only is this uncomfortable, but the bacteria can also cause infections around their genitals.

When to Worry

If your dog is experiencing pain when they urinate, or you find blood in their urine, they are likely suffering from a urinary tract infection or kidney disease. Once treated, you should find that the incontinence actually stops.

Lumps and Bumps

The strange little lumps that develop on or under your dog's skin can be quite distressing and, let's be honest, kind of gross. The good news is that they are completely natural and commonly show up as your dog ages. They are called lipomas and are caused by an accumulation of fatty cells. They are not cancerous and are unlikely to cause any pain.

How Can I Help?

There is typically nothing you can do to help with these growths. Removing them is not necessary as they don't pose a health risk. The most important thing to do is ensure that your dog is not scratching and opening them.

When to Worry

If these lumps continue to grow, become infected, or start to ooze, you should seek medical assistance. Your veterinarian will likely perform a biopsy to check if the growth is cancerous, and they may feel the need to remove it.

Bad Breath

Bad breath is generally caused by a gum infection or dead teeth. It is very common in aging dogs as their teeth begin to break, file down and decay with age. Injuries can also cause dental disease, and you may experience bad breath in younger dogs and puppies. This is very uncomfortable, and your dog is likely to experience pain when they eat. An infection can spread to the body and affect internal organs.

However, bad breath is not always a sign of dental conditions. Dogs can be pretty nasty, and for some reason, they love to eat disgusting things. If they have had access to garbage, carcasses, and even cat poop, they may be enjoying some hazardous snacks when you aren't looking.

How Can I Help?

Dental check! If your dog has broken teeth or a gum infection, take them to your veterinarian for a check-up and dental cleaning. In some cases, they may even remove the broken teeth. Once this is done, you will need to keep up with regular cleanings, which can be done at home.

If your dog is munching on disgusting items, make sure that they can no longer access them. Move your cat's litter box and ensure that all your bins are sealed.

When to Worry

If your dog passes the dental checks and is still experiencing bad breath, you will need to ask your veterinarian to investigate further. Diabetes, kidney disease, and liver disease can all cause strange-smelling breath. Knowing the other symptoms of these conditions can help you identify the cause.

Chapter 2:

Medical Conditions and Disease

If you are anything like me, I am sure you have been monitoring your dog carefully, and taking notes of every little sneeze and stumble. The looming, invisible threat of health complications can drive you over the edge. The thing is, these threats have always been there and while aging does come with its set of challenges, most medical issues that senior dogs experience are minor. It is not likely that your dog is going to suddenly become inflicted with a life-threatening medical condition.

However, that doesn't mean that you shouldn't be careful. Understanding the threats and how to spot them is the best way to prevent any complications. It is also the best way to decrease your anxiety! Always remember that your dog can pick up on your emotional state, and they will often mimic how you are feeling. In this chapter, we will discuss a variety of ailments, from acute to chronic, known to inflict senior dogs. While some of these are treatable at home, it is important to remember that you are not a veterinarian, and you can only do so much before you inflict more harm.

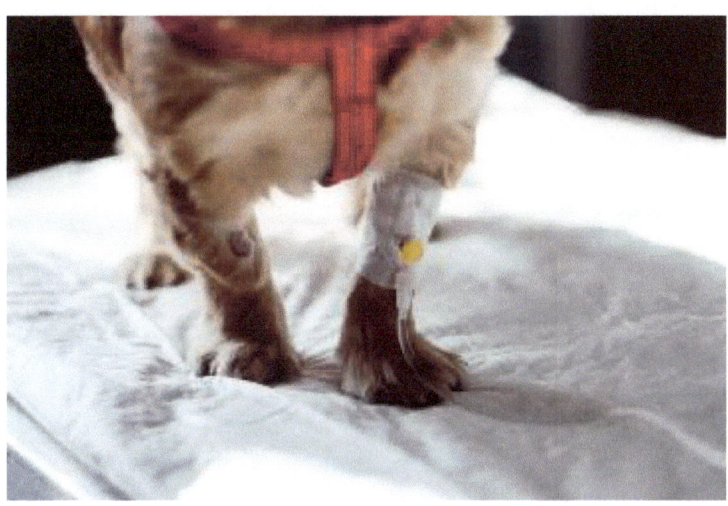

Treatment Options

There are a few different options you can choose from to treat your dog. However, before you attempt any home treatments, it is vital to understand the condition you are treating and the possible causes. Home treatments can mask symptoms that indicate a much more serious disease. Be smart, and work with your veterinarian to provide the best care for your pup.

Chronic vs. Acute

An acute illness infects the body quickly and the symptoms are seen within a few days. These types of illnesses usually last a week or two. Although the side effects may linger in the same way that you may recover from a cold, the cough may linger for a few weeks.

Chronic illnesses develop slowly and will typically worsen over time unless treated. These conditions last for months to years and, in some cases, a lifetime. Chronic conditions will often trigger acute ones. For example, a chronic allergy can cause acute abscesses if your dog scratches their skin open.

What Is Holistic Veterinary Care?

Holistic care is a form of healing that incorporates the body, mind, spirit, and environment. It is non-invasive and puts the dog's overall health and emotional well-being first. The goal is not to just treat the symptoms. It is finding the root cause of the illness and removing it to ensure that the condition does not worsen or recur. Holistic veterinarians will combine modern medicine with holistic treatments such as homeopathy, rehabilitation, dietary care, and pain management practices such as acupuncture.

Surgery may be performed to fix a broken leg, but this is just one symptom. Holistic care would incorporate rehabilitation to help your dog regain muscle. Homeopathy can help manage pain and muscle stiffness. Nutritional therapy can keep your dog's weight stable while they heal. Grooming can keep your dog's claws short, which will reduce pressure on the joints. As well as a change in your home environment can accommodate your dog's temporary disability and keep them comfortable.

What Is Homeopathic Treatment?

Homeopathy involves using natural animal, vegetable, or mineral substances to produce a remedy that relieves, treats, or cures a medical condition. The principle of homeopathy is, if a toxic amount of a substance causes dangerous health symptoms, then a much smaller amount of the same substance should be capable of healing those symptoms.

While most homeopathic treatments are safe, there can be adverse effects if you mix certain substances with medications. It is best to speak to your veterinarian first if your dog is suffering from a chronic condition. Dogs cannot always digest the same substances we do, so be sure to check the ingredients first and make sure they are safe. For acute conditions such as upset stomachs, sprains, and short stress periods, homeopathic remedies can work wonders!

Rescue Remedy is the absolute bee's knees. This is my all-time favorite homeopathic remedy, and if you don't have a bottle, I suggest you go get one right now. You can use it to calm your dog before or during a stressful event. I give my dog two drops before a thunderstorm, and he sleeps through it like a baby. It can also be used to treat pain and discomfort. It won't take the pain away completely, but it definitely makes it easier to handle.

Acute Conditions and Disease

Most acute conditions are easy to treat and even easier to prevent once you are aware of them. However, they should still be taken seriously, especially with senior dogs that may be suffering from other medical conditions.

Ear Infections

Ear infections can be very irritating. They are itchy and painful and can disorientate your dog. If not treated, the infection can actually cause permanent damage to your dog's hearing.

They are usually caused by bacteria that thrives in moisture and wax build-up. So, it is important to dry your dog's ears after they bathe or swim. Dogs with ear infections will often paw and scratch their ear repeatedly, sometimes to the point of scratching open the skin. The ear is typically red and swollen, and you may find discharge or crusting inside it. Depending on the extent of the infection, there will be a strong odor as well.

While this is considered an acute condition, some dogs may suffer from recurrent ear infections as a symptom of a chronic disorder. If you notice that this is happening, speak to your veterinarian.

Treatment

The best treatment will be a course of antibiotic ear drops. However, you can treat the secondary symptoms at home. Use a disinfectant to keep the outside of the ear clean and free from any discharge or crusting. This will help stop the itch, but make sure that you dry your dog's ear well and do not get any disinfectant in the ear canal.

If your dog has long fur, I strongly recommend that you trim the fur around and in the ears to keep them clean. Once the ear infection has subsided, you should routinely wash your dog's ears every month or so to prevent it from happening again.

Vomiting and Diarrhea

Vomiting is not always a serious problem. Eating too much too quickly is the most common cause. If your dog has eaten something mildly toxic like plastic or plants, their bodies will reject it, and they will vomit it up. One or two vomits in quick succession are nothing to worry about. However, if your dog is shaking, drooling, and vomiting up large amounts, they have likely eaten something very toxic. This is an emergency, and you will need to get to your vet as soon as possible.

Diarrhea is commonly due to a dietary change. This can occur if you move your dog onto new food too quickly or overload them with treats. Mildly toxic foods can also cause diarrhea. The worst thing in the world is cleaning up after a dog has stolen a piece of cake! These types of stomach upsets don't last long, and if your dog is acting normal and eating and drinking as usual, you can treat this at home.

If the diarrhea lasts for more than 24 hours or has any blood in it, you need to start worrying. This could be a sign of gastroenteritis, parasites, and toxicity. A dog suffering from these will be weak, dehydrated, and tired. They will completely lose their appetite and there will be a noticeable weight change.

Treatment

If the condition is severe, you will need to take your dog to a veterinarian immediately. They will be able to hydrate them, flush the body of any toxins and administer the correct medications.

In mild cases, you can treat it at home and the first step is to take away all food for 12 hours. Keep them warm and comfortable, and make sure they have access to plenty of water. Be prepared to clean up some potty mistakes, and lay down newspaper or potty pads if you aren't able to give them permanent access to the yard.

Rice water is absolutely wonderful for treating digestive disorders. It alleviates bloating and lines the stomach. You can make this by boiling 1 cup of white rice with 4 cups of water for 20 minutes. Strain the water out and allow it to cool before offering it to your dog. Giving them probiotics will also ease the upset.

For the next week, I suggest splitting up their meals into four portions. This will make sure that their stomachs are not overloaded, and they will be able to digest the food easier. Do not give them any treats, high-sugar foods, or human foods!

Constipation

For some reason, dogs truly love to eat things that they shouldn't. Toys, plants, dirt and even hair can cause an impaction in the intestine which leads to constipation. If you suspect that your dog has eaten a foreign object, head straight to your veterinarian. They will do an x-ray to see if they need to remove any squeaky toys from your dog's intestine!

Constipation can be caused by reasons apart from stupidity! A poor diet, dehydration and chronic medications can inflame the gut and make it difficult for your dog to digest and pass food. Dogs that suffer from food allergies are also likely to experience consistent constipation. Dogs that are constipated are often noticeably bloated and will lick their stomachs excessively to try and self-soothe.

Treatment

Do not give your dog any food for at least 12 hours, piling food on food will only make the situation worse. Provide them with plenty of water, probiotics, and electrolytes. Dog-safe laxatives and liquid paraffin will help to soften their stool, making it easier to pass. These can be purchased from your veterinarian, who will be able to direct you on the correct dosages. You may need to continue using laxatives and probiotics for a few days, even if your dog has started to potty normally.

If the constipation was not caused by an impaction, you will need to make a few lifestyle changes. A good quality diet that is high in fiber, plenty of clean water, and regular exercise is usually more than enough to prevent constipation!

Urinary Tract Infections

Dogs that are suffering from a bladder or urinary tract infection will struggle to urinate or whimper when they do. Their urine will have a pungent smell and, in severe cases, contain blood. Female dogs are more prone to infections, and they can be caused by bacteria, holding it in for too long, hormonal changes, and strong medications. If your dog suffers from a chronic condition such as diabetes or kidney disease, they will become more susceptible to bladder infections.

Treatment

There is no way around it, urinary tract infections will need to be treated with antibiotics! However, there are a few things you can do at home to support this treatment, relieve the symptoms, and prevent it from happening again. Clean, fresh water is critical. Frequent walks and potty breaks will prevent your dog from needing to hold it in for long periods of time.

Antioxidants, probiotics, and dog-friendly cranberry supplements will help to fight the infection and keep the stomach and bladder functioning normally. Antioxidant supplements have anti-inflammatory properties, which will ease the discomfort.

Stiffness and Sprains

Stiffness is not isolated to senior dogs, although they do experience it more often. This could be caused by a fall, a pulled muscle, too much exercise, or an injury. This can easily be treated at home, but if you are worried that there may be a more serious cause, take your pup to the veterinarian.

Treatment

If your pup has sprained their ankle, you can support it by wrapping it up with a bandage. Just make sure that the wrap is not too tight. It's best to remove the bandage at night and when it gets wet or dirty.

Homeopathic remedies such as Arnica or T-Relief work wonders for sore muscles! T-Relief can be purchased in tablet or drop form and is perfectly safe for dogs. Arnica can be toxic if ingested, so if you do use it, make sure to wrap it up with a bandage. When you remove the bandage, wash off the Arnica as well.

Epsom salts have anti-inflammatory properties and work well for treating muscular pain and swelling. Put half a cup into a warm bath and give your dog a soak for 5 to 10 minutes. You really don't want to soak your dog multiple times a day. Instead, soak a cloth in the warm mixture and hold it against the sore spot to provide relief.

Coughing

A cough or two is completely normal. Dogs will cough, hack or gag if they have eaten something that disagrees with them or have inhaled an irritating allergen. However, if your dog is coughing continuously, they may have kennel cough. Kennel cough is a relatively loose term that refers to a number of viral and bacterial infections that can inflame the throat. They will likely show other symptoms such as nasal discharge and gagging.

The main causes of it are parainfluenza and Bordetella. These are extremely contagious and any dog with symptoms should be isolated. Vaccinations are available for both of these illnesses. While it is mostly just annoying for healthy adult dogs, it can have serious health consequences for young puppies and seniors that have lowered or underdeveloped immune systems. This is just one of the reasons why it is so important to keep up with your dog's annual vaccinations.

If your dog only coughs during physical activity, you should visit your veterinarian immediately, as this could be due to a number of chronic medical conditions or tracheal collapse.

Treatment

There is no treatment for kennel cough, but there are ways to relieve the symptoms. Buy a humidifier, or sit with your dog in the bathroom while the shower is on. The steam will provide relief and loosen up mucus. Some children's cough syrups can also be given, but make sure you check with your vet to see which one is safe. The best treatment is to support their immune system. Create a comfortable, warm environment for them, with good food and loads of water. It's best to avoid strenuous exercise for a while, as this can put further strain on their lungs and throat.

It usually takes around three weeks for the cough to subside, but older dogs can take up to six weeks or more. Older dogs are also much more sensitive to the cold and need to be monitored carefully, as kennel cough can lead to pneumonia.

Parasites

External parasites like ticks and fleas are easy enough to see. Mites, on the other hand, are microscopic. They cause the same symptoms, and you will notice that your dog scratches obsessively, chews their paws, and rubs their face and ears. Most mites are harmless but incredibly irritating and if not treated, your dog will begin to lose fur and develop wounds from excessive scratching.

Sarcoptic mites are the most dangerous as they cause mange, which is a severe skin infection. Dogs with mange will lose all their fur and their skin will be covered in sores and scabs. This is highly contagious and can spread to other mammals, birds, and even reptiles.

At some point, your dog will get internal parasites. It is inevitable! These parasites can be picked up from soil, dog parks, feces, and carcasses. If you enjoy giving your dog a kiss before bed, you should probably be dewormed too! In healthy dogs, these parasites aren't too dangerous, and you can treat them easily at home. In young puppies, seniors, or immune-compromised dogs, parasites can turn deadly.

Dogs that have worms will often scoot by rubbing their rumps on the ground. In more serious cases, you may notice a drastic drop in weight, dehydration, and blood and worms in their feces. If the infection has gotten to this point, it is best to get your dog to a veterinarian.

Treatment

There are a variety of different products on the market to kill internal and external parasites. Some products kill both in one go! However, you will notice that there is a big price difference between them. Regular dewormers will kill hookworms, roundworms, and tapeworms. Regular external parasite medications will only kill ticks and fleas.

I recommend purchasing one of the most specialized products at least once a year. These will also kill off ear and sarcoptic mites, heartworm, and whipworms.

Dewormers should be given every 3 to 6 months, depending on your dogs' exposure to contaminated soils and other dogs. Tick and flea medications are given every 1 to 3 months, depending on the brand. Avoid using parasite dips! These are very harsh on the skin and can cause severe reactions if ingested.

Abscesses

Abscesses are sneaky little pockets of puss that develop under the skin. This is generally due to a bacterial infection caused by a bite or wound. It can be difficult to see at first, but as the pus collects, the lump will become more prominent. They become increasingly painful as they grow and can develop anywhere on the body and inside the mouth. If left untreated, the infection will likely spread and cause necrosis and organ damage. In some cases, the abscess will burst by itself when it grows too large; however, if the puss is not completely drained, it will come back.

Treatment

There is no fun way to say it, an abscess has to be drained. In some cases, your veterinarian might find it necessary to lance it to get the bulk of the pus out. This typically leaves a large pocket under the skin which is susceptible to further infection. You will need to flush this pocket out every day to remove any debris, pus, and dirt.

Do not try to lance an abscess at home! It is incredibly painful, and you can cause your dog more pain. If you are dealing with a small abscess and your dog is not showing any other signs of infection, you can treat it with Epsom salts. Mix some in warm water and soak a cotton cloth. Hold the cloth on the abscess until it cools and then repeat it. This will help to open up the abscess and it will drain itself. Continue doing this a few times a day for the next week to completely clear it out.

If your dog shows any sign of infection, your veterinarian will need to prescribe a course of antibiotics to treat the bacterial infection.

Chronic Conditions and Disease

Chronic conditions should be taken seriously, regardless of your dog's age. The symptoms may not look as severe when your dog is young and full of energy, but as they get older, the condition will worsen if not treated. If your dog is showing any of the below symptoms, it is time to visit your veterinarian!

Obesity

Obesity and arthritis are the two most common chronic conditions seen in senior dogs. It is no surprise that the two are often linked. Stiffness and pain in the joints make your dog reluctant to exercise, which causes weight gain. A heavier body puts immense strain on these already painful joints, making it even more difficult to exercise.

Obesity, in general, has a considerable impact on your dog's overall health. It places strain on the organs, which exacerbates chronic conditions, and it can lead to diabetes.

Treatment

Obesity requires a strict diet change and exercise routine. It can take months to get your dog's weight back to a healthy level, and it is up to you to stay consistent. Treatments will be discussed more in-depth in the following chapters.

Diabetes

Diabetes can be separated into Type 1 and Type 2. Type 1 diabetes occurs when the body is unable to produce insulin. Type 2 diabetes occurs when the body is unable to use insulin correctly.

When your dog eats, the food is broken down and the nutrients are separated in the digestive system. One of these nutrients is glucose, which is carried to cells in the body by the hormone insulin. If the body is unable to produce insulin or use it efficiently, the blood sugar levels will spike and cause hyperglycemia.

This will cause a change in appetite, weight loss, excessive thirst, and dehydration. Most dogs will have strange, sweet-smelling breath, and you may notice that they urinate more often and develop urinary infections easily.

While there is no exact cause, it has been linked with autoimmune disorders, obesity, and even some chronic medications. Some breeds such as Poodles, Dachshunds, and Miniature Schnauzers are also more prone to developing diabetes as they age.

Treatment

Dogs that have diabetes will require regular insulin injections to keep their blood sugar levels in check. However, this is not enough to keep them healthy. Obesity is known to exacerbate diabetic systems, so it is important to feed your dog a healthy diet and continue with regular exercise. Avoid treats and foods that are high in sugar, and increase the amount of fiber in their diet. Fiber will slow down the absorption of sugar from food, which will keep your dog's blood sugar levels from spiking.

Arthritis

As your dog ages, their joints deteriorate, and they have an increased chance of developing arthritis. It can affect one or all of their limbs and is more likely to occur if they have suffered a previous injury.

You may find that your dog struggles to jump the heights that they once could. They struggle to get up and lay down without shaking and in some cases, they may develop a limp. These signs are particularly noticeable in cold and damp weather.

While it is quite distressing, it is not uncommon and around 80% of dogs will develop arthritis in their senior years.

Treatment

Strenuous and spontaneous exercise should be avoided at all costs. That means no more jumping in and out of the car! Short, slow walks will help them to stretch out and keep fit without the risk of injury. Foods and supplements that promote joint health and mobility are great options for relieving discomfort and combating weight gain.

Sweaters, socks, warm blankets, and heated beds can help alleviate joint discomfort during cold weather.

If your dog has developed a severe limp or struggles to stand up without falling, it is time to worry! A veterinarian will be able to assess the extent of the arthritis through an x-ray and provide you with an appropriate treatment plan. In most cases, you will be given a prescription for pain management medication, which will help take the edge off.

Allergies

Allergies can be caused by numerous factors. Environmental allergies are most common and include allergens such as pollen, grass, mold, and dust mites. These allergies are more likely to flare up in spring and summer. While you may see more conventional signs such as runny nose, watery eyes, and sneezing, these allergies mainly affect the skin. Dogs will often rub their faces, or bodies against the ground or grass to stop the itch. The worst itch occurs in the paws, and dogs will sit and lick and chew them for hours on end. Excessive licking and chewing on a certain spot can cause open wounds, fur loss, and inflammation.

Food allergies are a little less common but still account for 10% of allergic reactions. Dogs will display the same itchy symptoms, but can also experience bloating, constipation, vomiting, and diarrhea. The most common food allergens are beef, chicken, fish, dairy, soy, gluten, and general additives.

Treatment

Environmental allergies are very difficult to treat. The best thing that you can do is ensure that the house is clean and free of dust, mites, and mold. If there are specific plants that are causing the reaction, it is best to remove them from the yard. Pollen and grass allergies can't be cured, but they can be controlled by using antihistamines during spring and summer. If you suspect your dog is suffering from food allergies, you will need to change them to a hypoallergenic diet. These are free of common allergens and safe for the stomach.

Regular baths with a sensitive shampoo will relieve the itch and reduce any inflammation. Oatmeal has anti-inflammatory properties and works brilliantly for inflamed skin. Grind some up into a powder and mix it with water to make a paste. You can pack this paste onto any inflamed areas to soothe them. This works best for paws, and you can push the paste in between their paw pads. It is completely safe to eat, and your dog will have a great time licking it off themselves!

If your pup has dry, flaking skin from allergies, rub them down with coconut oil. It's edible, relieves itches, moisturizes the skin, and promotes beautiful soft fur growth. You can't go wrong.

Cancer

Cancer is terrifying and for many owners, this is the last diagnosis they ever want to hear. However, cancer is not always fatal, and many treatments are available to improve your dog's quality of life . This, of course, depends on the type of cancer and how far it has spread.

As your dog ages, the odds of abnormal cell growth increase. These cells surround and affect tissue, muscle, and organs. Localized cancers such as tumors are confined to specific locations in the body. Generalized cancers can spread throughout the body and damage everything in their path. There is no single cause for the growth of cancerous cells. A variety of environmental, genetic, and dietary factors can be responsible. Breeds such as golden retrievers, boxers, beagles, and Burmese mountain dogs are more prone to developing cancer.

The symptoms your dog displays will depend heavily on which part of the body is impacted. Lethargy, weight loss, muscle weakness, swelling, and lack of appetite are common symptoms, but these are not enough for a full diagnosis.

Yearly blood tests are vital for senior dogs as they will allow your veterinarian to pick up inflammation, infection, and abnormal hormone levels. X-rays, ultrasounds, and other tests need to be done before a diagnosis is made.

Treatment

Treatment will depend on the location and severity of the cancer. Early detection is key, as the further the cancer spreads, the more difficult it is to fight. Most localized cancers and tumors can be surgically removed. Chemotherapy and radiation are used for more generalized cancers, especially ones that affect internal organs.

However, when choosing a treatment option, it is important to consider your dog's age and their strength. A younger, healthy dog is strong enough to go through chemotherapy with a good chance of survival and recovery.

Elderly dogs will likely be too weak and in these cases, your veterinarian will suggest palliative care. This involves treating the symptoms and managing the pain to make your dog as comfortable as possible during their last few months or years.

Hypothyroidism

The thyroid is located next to the windpipe. This incredibly important gland releases hormones that control the metabolism. If too many hormones are released, hyperthyroidism occurs, and the metabolism is elevated. If the gland isn't able to produce enough, hypothyroidism occurs. This slows down the metabolism immensely. Dogs suffering from it will experience a noticeable increase in weight, yet no increase in their appetite.

The skin will often be dry and flaky, and their fur will become dry with dull fur. You may also notice bald patches along the body. As the condition continues, your dog will likely become sluggish and lethargic and show a reluctance to exercise. The chance of ear infections, high cholesterol, and muscle loss will also increase the longer it is left untreated.

This condition is usually caused by autoimmune diseases such as lymphocytic thyroiditis. While it isn't common, it is known to affect Labradors, Irish setters, boxers, and dachshunds.

Treatment

If your dog is displaying any of these symptoms, your veterinarian will take a blood test to confirm the diagnosis. Unfortunately, this condition is not curable, but replacement hormones can be given. This is a lifelong treatment, but it allows your dog to live a happy, long life.

To find the correct dose, the veterinarian will inject your dog with the thyroid hormone and then conduct a blood test a few hours later. This allows them to determine if the dose given was enough to stabilize their thyroid hormone levels. A blood test will need to be done every six months to monitor these levels and the dose will be adjusted accordingly.

Chapter 3:

Preventive Veterinary Care

Now that you are aware of the possible medical issues your dog may experience, it is time to learn how to prevent them from happening in the first place! Prevention is achieved by using every available resource in your arsenal, from dietary care and exercise to regular grooming. However, the most important and reliable resource you have is your veterinarian.

Some dogs are masters at hiding pain or illness and while you know your dog best, a veterinarian will be able to pick up on subtle symptoms that you may have missed. It is recommended that dogs over the age of seven undertake two health checks a year to ensure that any changes in their condition are noted. From there, your veterinarian will be able to guide you through treatments and show you the necessary changes that need to be made at home.

Let's take a look at what actually happens during these health checks, and what your veterinarian will be looking for.

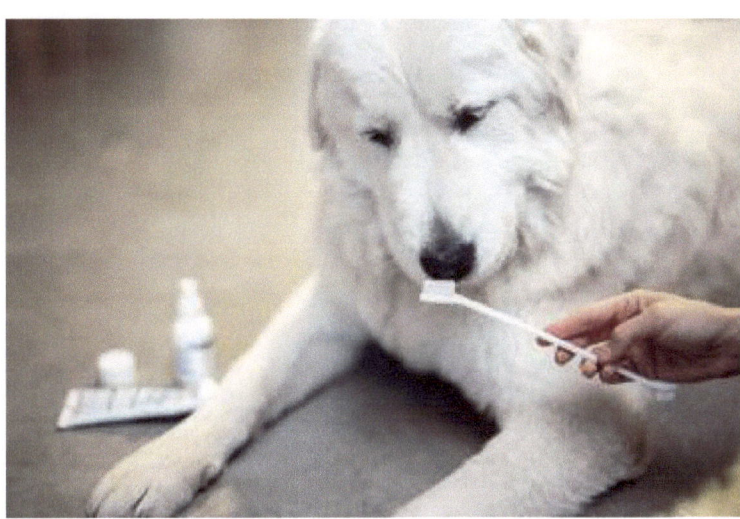

Understanding Your Breed

For centuries, we have selectively bred dogs with specific genes to produce new and exciting breeds that possess unique physical, behavioral, and emotional traits. The problem is that we have allowed a couple of bad genes to slip through as well. These are responsible for the variety of genetic medical disorders that we see today.

Genetic disorders are commonly associated with purebred dogs, as mixed breeds have a much lower chance of two parents sharing the same recessive gene. Reputable breeders will ensure that their mating pairs are healthy and free of these genes. This is why purchasing a puppy from a breeder can be so expensive.

Backyard breeders and "puppy mills" value profit over their dogs. They can cut down costs by ignoring the breeding guidelines and voiding health checks and DNA sampling. Dogs from the same litter will often be interbred to produce as many puppies as possible for a much cheaper price. This rise in inbreeding caused an inevitable wave of dogs born with predispositions to medical conditions and sadly, it still continues.

Breed History

Reputable breeders will provide you with medical records and health certificates to prove that the puppies are healthy and possess no recessive genes. If you have not been provided with one or if you have rescued a purebred dog that has no history, it is time for some tests! Your veterinarian will identify specific worrisome genes through a series of blood tests. This can be costly, but it is worth it for some piece of mind.

Common Genetic and Chronic Disorders

Degenerative Myelopathy is a disease that causes the nerves in the spinal cord to deteriorate. This leads to weakness in the hind legs and, in severe cases, incontinence and paralysis. German shepherds are at the highest risk, but Bernese mountain dogs, boxers, and spaniels are also susceptible. Unfortunately, there is no way to prevent or treat this disease. However, the gene can be detected through blood tests, which allows you enough time to prepare your dog for it.

Dilated Cardiomyopathy is a disease that causes the heart muscles to weaken. Dobermans, boxers, Great Danes, and Irish setters are all high-risk breeds. Unfortunately, there is no way to test for this gene and therefore no way to predict it. While it cannot be cured, there are several supportive medications that can be used to provide your dog with a longer, more comfortable life.

Brachycephalic Syndrome is a respiratory deformity. This occurs in breeds such as bulldogs, pugs, and Boston terriers, which have rounded heads and flat faces. As a result of the much shorter snout, these dogs often have slit-like nostrils and a narrow trachea, which makes it incredibly difficult to breathe. This can be especially dangerous during exercise, stress, and hot days. As your dog's breathing increases and they pant heavily, the trachea may collapse.

English bulldogs are unfortunately the most susceptible due to an increase in inbreeding, and many require surgery at a young age to correct it.

Chondrodysplasia affects long, short breeds such as dachshunds and basset hounds. Due to their significantly short leg bones, their joints end up taking a lot of strain, which can cause severe arthritis as they age. Their spine is disproportionately long, and their legs are unable to properly support it. This puts stress on the spinal discs, which can lead to injury and disc disease.

Hip Dysplasia is one of the most common and well-known genetic disorders. It impacts large and giant breeds such as German shepherds, Labradors, Great Danes, and Saint Bernards being the most susceptible. These breeds grow rapidly. Sometimes, too quickly and the increase in muscle mass and weight puts too much strain on their still-developing skeleton. The hips and shoulders take the brunt of this weight and will shift and deform to accommodate it.

If it is caught early enough, there are surgeries that can be done to reshape the hip. Sadly, it is usually diagnosed too late and while surgeries are still available, the dog will likely end up suffering from severe arthritis.

These are just some of the many genetic disorders that can impact different breeds. However, it is important to remember that just because these breeds have a predisposition, there is no guarantee that they will develop these conditions.

Annual Veterinary Visits

Don't be a vet hopper! Going to the vet is scary enough, especially if your dog has had a painful experience there. Getting them comfortable with one veterinarian at one facility can greatly decrease their stress response.

Sticking with one veterinarian allows them to develop a good relationship with your dog and become familiar with their behaviors and physical condition. This will make it much easier for them to pick up on behavioral changes that indicate injury or illness. By using the same veterinary practice, you can rest assured that they will have all of your dog's medical information on file. If your veterinarian is ever away, the next one on duty will be able to take over without any hassle.

Annual Physicals

Regardless of age, your dog should go for a full check-up once a year. As they age, you will likely need to increase this to every six months. During these check-ups, your veterinarian will ask you if there have been any changes to your lifestyle and if you have noticed a change in your dogs' behavior, diet, and overall health. It is important to be completely honest, don't try to hide any embarrassing mistakes!

They will then begin a head-to-tail examination. Your veterinarian will check your dog's eyes, ears, mouth, and teeth. They will stretch out their legs to check their mobility and feel and prod along their stomachs to check for bloat or compaction.

Senior check-ups will take a little longer as your veterinarian will focus on identifying any age-related conditions. These may include arthritis, cancers, infections, and eyesight and hearing loss. If they do find anything peculiar, further tests will be done to confirm the diagnosis.

Annual Vaccinations

So many owners stop vaccinating their dogs as they grow older, which simply doesn't make sense! Senior dogs are much more susceptible to viruses and disease due to their lowered immune system. These annual vaccinations protect your dog from distemper, parvovirus, parainfluenza, and hepatitis. All of these are extremely contagious, and can be deadly for dogs with weakened or underdeveloped immune systems.

Annual Procedures

Your veterinarian will likely recommend several procedures to be done on a yearly basis to monitor the internal health of your dog. These can be quite costly and if money is tight, you should request that only the most important ones are done.

X-rays will be done to check the health of your dog's bones, joints, and the presence of arthritis. If your dog has been struggling with digestive or respiratory problems, your vet will likely take a gut and chest x-ray as well.

A complete blood count and chemical screening will be done to monitor how your dog's kidneys, liver, and heart are functioning. This will help your veterinarian to pick up on any cancers, infections, and disorders that may be hiding.

If your pup has not been dewormed, your veterinarian will do a fecal flotation, which will help them to pick up any signs of internal parasites.

Keep All Your Pet Documents!

This is a no-brainer. Get yourself a file and store all of your dog's medical information. This should include anything and everything from adoption and breeder certificates and vaccination records to x-rays and test results. If your dog has suffered from any injuries or illnesses, keep a record of the treatments and medications they received. Make sure to keep a list of allergies they may have as well. If, for whatever reason, you need to change to a new veterinarian, you will be able to provide them with your dog's full medical history.

I also recommend making a separate emergency folder. This should include your personal information, your veterinarian's contact details, and your dogs' information. Be sure to add in a list of any medical conditions and medications that your dog may be on. When you go away, you can hand this folder over to whoever is caring for your pup!

Emergency Care

Ideally, you want to avoid dealing with any emergencies. Through preventative care, you should be able to catch any condition early enough to treat it in time. However, accidents do happen and while you can't prevent them, you can be prepared for them.

If you don't have a pet first aid kit already, it is time to make one. You may never need it, but it certainly does come in handy the day that you do. This will give you the ability to treat minor wounds at home and administer emergency first aid to stabilize your dog until you can get to your veterinarian.

Your emergency information folder should be kept with your kit at all times, and I strongly recommend that you get a dog first aid guide. You can purchase them or source them online for free. These short pamphlets contain detailed instructions with pictures of how to administer CPR as well as how to deal with choking, poisoning, seizures, and more!

Pet First Aid Kit

These are some of the most important items to have. Excluding any medications that your veterinarian has given you, of course.

- Hydrogen peroxide—A fantastic wound cleaner that can be used to flush out dirt and debris.

- Antibiotic ointment—This ointment protects wounds and scratches from becoming infected. Depending on which one you get, it can also ease swelling and itchiness caused by allergies and insect bites.

- Styptic powder—Stops excessive bleeding by causing the blood to clot. Great for nips during grooming and claw cutting.

- Antiseptic wipes—It's always best to keep your dog clean. If they have scratched or injured themselves, you will need to remove any dirt around the wound immediately. If you don't, it can cause infection!

- Gauze—Stock up on a variety of sizes and lengths. These are great for stopping bleeding and wrapping up a wound to protect it from dirt. Use it to strap up a sprained leg and a makeshift muzzle if needed.

- Tape—You will need flexible tape to keep your gauze and bandages fixed in place. I prefer to use non-adhesive ones because the glues can get stuck in your dog's fur, making it painful to remove.

- Thermometer]—For doggy use only! This is one of the most important first-aid tools you can have. If you are ever worried that your dog is ill, take their temperature. A healthy temperature is between 101 and 102.5 °F. Anything higher usually indicates infection, while a low temperature indicates hypothermia.

- Gloves—Keep a pair of sterile latex gloves in your first aid kit. You should always wear these if you are dealing with open wounds, as you want to avoid spreading bacteria. If you don't have any, be sure to thoroughly wash your hands.

- Scissors—When is a good pair of scissors not handy?

- Syringes—Keep a couple of different-sized syringes in your kit. These are great for measuring out and administering medications and can be used for flushing out wounds.

- Tweezers—Tweezers are handy for removing splinters, ticks, bee stings, and any dirt or debris from wounds.

- Flashlight—A flashlight allows you to inspect hard-to-see spots on your dog's body. It's especially helpful for inspecting their mouth and paws.

- Towel or blanket—A good towel is extremely versatile. You can use it as a ground cover to keep your pup off the floor. Or wrap them up in it to keep them warm and calm. It can even be used as a makeshift tourniquet and an absorbent pad to stop bleeding.

- Soft fabric muzzle—Dogs that are in a high-stress mode after an emotionally distressing event are more likely to bite. A soft muzzle can help to keep them calm and prevent them from injuring you and themselves.

- Extra leash—It's not uncommon for dogs to snap their leash when they panic. You may just be unable to find your usual one. Regardless, having an extra one will provide you with immediate control over your pup and prevent further injuries.

Chapter 4:

Healthy Diet, Healthy Dog!

Food is your body's primary energy source, you use the nutrients and minerals from it to grow, maintain and heal. This is why it makes perfect sense to provide puppies with protein and calcium-rich foods. As our puppies grow, we swap them onto healthy maintenance food to keep their health in check. Yet, when it comes to senior dogs, a change in food is almost always overlooked!

As our dogs age, their teeth will often file down, break, or become brittle, which can make it much harder to chew the larger pieces of food they are used to. If your dog is struggling to eat, they will likely lose weight. Soft food is a great solution to this problem as it is much easier to chew. The only issue here is that many owners don't know how to correctly portion canned food, and too much of a good thing can cause excessive weight gain and plaque build-up.

Thankfully, there are plenty of dog foods out there that have been designed specifically for different-sized senior dogs. These foods contain the vital nutrients, at the right levels, that an old dog needs to thrive while still maintaining a balanced weight.

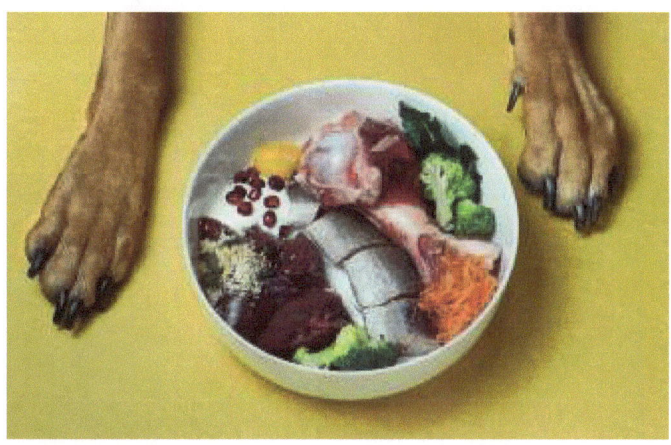

Should I Change My Dog's Food?

Yes, you definitely should. Specialized foods will help control medical conditions and remedy weight fluctuations. However, you shouldn't wait until these conditions arise. Moving over to an old dog diet when your dog first enters their senior years will promote a healthy immune system and prevent some medical conditions from occurring in the first place.

Dental Concerns

There is nothing worse than trying to eat hard foods with a sore mouth. Broken teeth and gum disease are the usual suspects. If you haven't been looking after your dog's teeth or if they like to eat or munch on hard items and bones, you can expect a tooth extraction or two.

Smaller-sized kibble can help tremendously and if your dog still struggles to chew, you can use hot water to soften it. I like to mix in a hot gravy to make my own style of soft canned food.

Canned foods are great, the small soft pieces are easy on the mouth and are highly digestible. If you want to swap over to soft foods permanently, you need to do your research! Cheap, store-bought brands generally lack vital nutrients and most are packed with sugars and fat. Opt for veterinary standard foods that are designed for senior dogs.

Weight Concerns

A drop in weight is pretty scary, but it is relatively easy to fix once you know the cause. Getting treatment for any medical conditions that are contributing to the weight loss is the first step. Thereafter, a change in diet, an extra meal a day and some added supplements will get your dog back to a healthy weight.

An increase in weight is a lot more difficult to fix. It happens gradually, so most owners don't notice until it is severe. Typically, this is due to overfeeding, excessive treats, and a lack of exercise. Basically, this comes down to you. However, some breeds are more prone to obesity than others. Pugs, golden retrievers and basset hounds are at the most risk.

The Dangers of Obesity

Obesity is a gateway to numerous health issues. A heavier body is heavier on the joints and if your dog is suffering from arthritis, this can be extremely painful. The extra fat will collect around organs, placing immense strain on them. This can lead to liver and kidney damage, diabetes, and difficulty breathing.

With all this added discomfort, it is perfectly understandable why your dog is reluctant to exercise! The problem is, with this reluctance, your dog is bound to gain even more weight. If not remedied quickly, it can cut your dog's lifespan down by up to two years.

Meal Planning

Correct food portions and meal planning is your first step to controlling weight gain. You can cut down a good number of pounds, which will ease the strain on your dog's body, allowing them to get back into an exercise routine comfortably.

Firstly, cut down on the treats that are full of sugars and fat, and stop giving your dog any human foods! Dogs aren't able to digest the same foods that we do.

Next, purchase food that suits your dog's needs. Metabolic and weight control foods are specially formulated for this issue. However, you can use normal senior dog foods if you learn to portion them correctly.

Good dog foods will come with a feeding chart that indicates the correct portion sizes for your dog's weight and activity level. For example, the chart may tell you that a 20-pound, low-activity dog should be fed 5 ounces a day. However, a 20-pound, high-activity dog should be fed 6 ounces. This is because high-activity dogs are burning off the calories much quicker.

If you know that your dog should be fed 6 ounces a day, split this into 2 portions and feed them 3 ounces for breakfast and 3 ounces for dinner.

Weight Loss Management

Speak to your veterinarian about what your dog's ideal weight should be. You can then work at gradually reducing their meal portions until they reach this weight. Graduality is key! Starving your dog is cruel and can lead to a whole new list of health issues.

If your dog weighs 20 pounds, feed them the recommended amount for a 19-pound dog. Once they get to 19 pounds, feed them the amount for an 18-pound dog. Continue feeding like this until your dog reaches their ideal weight.

There is no doubt that you will start to see improvement in their energy levels immediately. Be sure not to revert to old habits. Just because your dog is now at a stable weight does not mean that you can start giving them tons of treats and ice cream again.

Choosing Your Food

Your choice of food is going to depend greatly on the size of your dog, their breed, and what medical conditions they may be suffering from. It can be quite stressful to choose the right one, and it is always best to chat with your veterinarian if you need help. Senior dogs are more prone to sensitivities, so it is important to introduce new foods gradually and monitor them. If they show signs of allergy or digestive issues, you will need to rethink your food choice.

Adult vs. Senior Foods

Puppies need to do a great deal of growing in the first year or two of their lives. During this time, it is important to provide them with vitamins and minerals that promote healthy bone growth and digestive care. Puppy foods will have a higher fat and protein content to compensate for their active lifestyle.

Once your dog reaches adulthood, they should switch to a maintenance diet. These foods are generally lower in fat and carbohydrates, and the vitamin and mineral content will shift. Calcium and phosphorus content, which promote bone growth and health, will be considerably less in adult foods because your dog is no longer growing. Overall, this diet is designed to promote general health and maintain your dog's metabolism and immune system.

Senior dog diets contain much less fat. This is because old dogs' metabolisms slow down considerably, and they cannot process and expend the amount of energy they get from their food. Without this adjustment, old dogs are likely to gain weight and can suffer from constipation or diarrhea. The protein content in this food is much higher as it helps the body to maintain muscle mass.

Once again, the vitamin and mineral content will shift. Most senior foods will contain new supplements such as glucosamine for joint health and fish oils to combat allergies and skin conditions.

Breed-Specific Foods

Some pure breeds are more prone to genetic disorders and require specialized diets to keep them fit and healthy. This mainly includes small and toy breeds such as Yorkshire Terriers, Chihuahuas, and Pugs and giant breeds such as the Great Dane. However, specialized diets are also recommended for Labradors and German Shepherds who are prone to hip dysplasia.

Medical Foods

Let's face it, you will likely end up purchasing prescription food for your senior. These foods are specifically designed with a variety of nutrients and ingredients to combat specific medical conditions.

Mobility foods are great for dogs that are suffering from stiff joints and arthritis. They include Omega-3 fatty acids and antioxidants, which relieve inflammation. As well as glucosamine and chondroitin, which promote healthy joints.

Hypoallergenic food can be used for seniors that suffer from skin and food allergies. These avoid common allergens such as grains, soy, dairy, and artificial additives.

If your dog struggles with digestive issues, easily digestible metabolic foods are the best choice. These have a high fiber content and contain probiotics and flaxseed oils, which protect the stomach.

Weight control foods are ideal for obese seniors. They have a low fat, high fiber, high-protein content with an overall low-calorie count. This food has to be paired with regular exercise to work efficiently.

Each of these specialized foods comes in different sizes to suit small, medium, or large dogs. If your dog struggles to eat kibble, you can opt for the soft, canned options. If your dog suffers from two or more conditions, it is best to chat with your veterinarian. They will be able to direct you on which food is best and which ones you could potentially mix.

Clean Water

Keeping your dog's food and water bowls clean is absolutely vital. Your senior pup's immune system is not what it used to be, and bacteria build-up can have dire consequences. E. coli, yeast, mold, and salmonella can all grow in moist, dirty bowls. This is more common in plastic bowls, which may also release a variety of chemicals when left to decay. Stainless steel or glass bowls are best. They are easy to clean and reduce the risk of bacteria build-up.

Food bowls should be washed after every meal, and water bowls should be changed twice a day. Change the water again if it has been contaminated by debris, food, and, if you have a water lover, dirty paws. I like to have two sets of bowls and while one is in use, the other is in the dishwasher.

Helpful Vitamins and Supplements

Vitamins and supplements can make a considerable improvement to your senior dog's quality of life. However, it is important to use them correctly and not overload your dog's system.

All supplements will come with instructions that will direct you on how much to give your dog per day. Make sure to stick to these guidelines! Mixing up several different supplements can be quite dangerous. If you feel this is necessary, it is best to chat with your veterinarian first. They can help you decide what is best for your dog, which supplements are vital, and which ones you can ditch.

Multivitamins

Multivitamins are a great, all-around supplement that can be given to dogs of any age. These contain basic minerals, vitamins, and oils that promote overall body and mind health. Vitamins A, B, and E are added to support the brain, heart, and skin. While minerals such as calcium, iron, zinc, and copper support bone, blood, and organ health.

Geriatric Vitamins

These vitamins are created specifically for senior dogs. They contain vital minerals and vitamins that aren't usually found in standard multivitamins. Biotin and Omega oils promote skin and fur health and relieve general skin conditions. Vitamin C and E are natural antioxidants, and vitamin B improves the immune system. Most senior vitamins will also contain glucosamine, which reduces inflammation and relieves arthritis symptoms.

Medical Supplements

If your dog needs extra help with a specific condition, it is best to choose an appropriate medical supplement. These will contain specialized oils, vitamins, and minerals that are proven to combat the effects of certain conditions.

As with any supplement, the cheaper you go, the less effective they will be. Purchasing top-quality products will ensure that your dog's condition improves and reduce the chance of side effects.

Antioxidants

All of our bodies contain pesky little molecules called free radicals which directly damage the cells that form our organs, muscles, and tissues. They can form during periods of stress, illness, and dietary changes, but become more prominent when the body ages. Antioxidants such as vitamins A, C, and E, magnesium, and zinc fight off free radicals and support the immune system to prevent illness.

Joint Care

Joint supplements will greatly improve your dog's overall mobility. This supplement generally comes in a liquid form, which is easy to measure and pour onto your dog's breakfast. It contains glucosamine and chondroitin. Both of these ingredients are scientifically proven to increase the production of joint fluid. This fluid is responsible for the health of the cartilage that covers the joints. Most joint supplements will also contain Omega-3 oil, which reduces inflammation and pain.

Digestive Care

The stomach is full of good bacteria that help us to digest our food. As your dog ages or becomes ill, these bacteria are lost, and they will start to experience stomach upsets. Probiotics will reintroduce these bacteria and restore normal gut health. Digestive supplements are a little more advanced. They have a high fiber content and contain probiotics and digestive enzymes, which help the body to efficiently absorb nutrients.

Digestive supplements and probiotics are completely safe in the correct dosage and can be given to your dog for an extended period of time.

Allergy Care

Allergy supplements will generally contain probiotics and digestive enzymes to help with food-related allergies. Omega-3, 6, and 9 fatty acids and biotin help to keep the skin healthy and combat the effects of skin-related allergies. Good quality allergy supplements will contain quercetin and turmeric. These are natural antihistamines and anti-inflammatories, which will fight off the cause of the allergy.

Chapter 5:

Keeping Fit (Slowly)

Exercising your senior dog is just as important as exercising a puppy. Regular movement is vital for digestive health and without it, your dog can become prone to obesity and constipation. However, it is not only the body that ends up suffering. Anxiety and boredom-related behavioral problems are often linked directly to a lack of regular exercise and outdoor exposure.

It can be tricky and even a little scary trying to exercise a senior dog, especially ones that have existing medical conditions. The last thing you want to do is force them into a situation where they could get hurt. The key is choosing an exercise that suits your dog and their condition and then keeping the sessions short and sweet. Ten minutes of exercise a day is better than none! Let's take a look at some age-friendly exercises and how you can adapt them to suit your dog's needs.

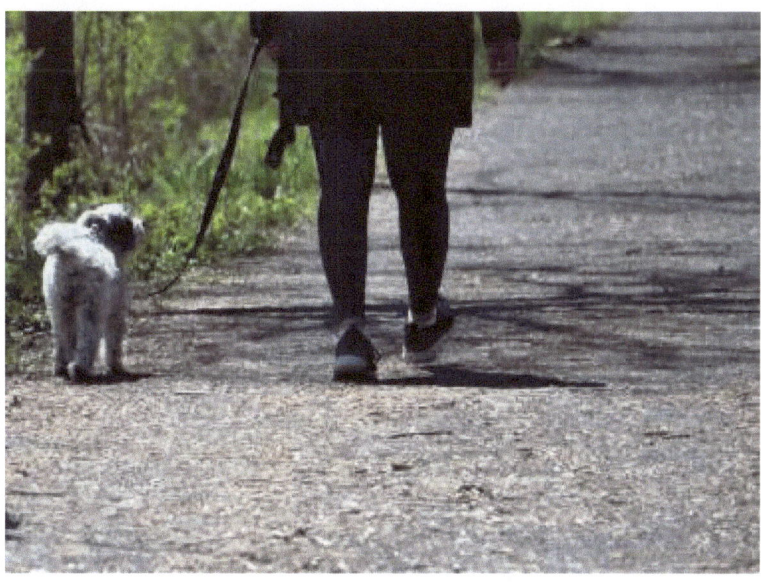

Knowing When To Slow Down

Dogs live for the now, not for the future! If all your senior wants to do is eat and nap all day, they will. If they feel like sprinting around the house, they will. If it doesn't hurt right now, why would it later? They may not understand, but we certainly do, and it is our responsibility to protect and care for them. Even when it means stopping them from having fun.

Are You Listening To Your Dog?

It can be pretty confusing trying to communicate with your dog. They send out such mixed signals! It is concerning when your dog limps their way back to you after fetching the ball. Except, their tail is wagging, and they have a huge goofy grin on their face as they wait for you to throw it again. Maybe they are actually okay? Think of it this way, if your toddler throws up after eating too many sweets, but then continues to eat more, would you let them? Always focus on what their bodies are telling you.

Abnormal Behaviors

Your dog will display numerous abnormal behaviors, which should tell you that they need to stop. By ignoring these red flags, you are guaranteeing injury. The most obvious sign will be slowing down by themselves or reluctance to partake in any physical activities. This is not necessarily due to injury or pain. Your dog's body just can't keep up, and they are likely to tire out quicker.

Appetite changes and excessive drinking should always be taken seriously. This is commonly caused by illness, digestive problems, or dental pain.

Excessive panting and drooling are often signs of heat stroke, stress, and dehydration. Dehydration is not necessarily caused by a lack of available water or exposure to heat. It can be caused by illness or kidney disease.

Disorientation, bumping into objects and irritability can indicate several health conditions. If your dog is displaying any of the behaviors above, during or after exercising, you should stop your routine completely. Your veterinarian will be able to diagnose the cause and treat it if necessary. Once your pup has recovered, introduce exercise slowly.

Signs and Symptoms of Pain and Injury

If your dog begins to favor one leg over the other during exercise or play time, it is best to stop the activity immediately. This could just be from stiffness or a bit of weakness. However, if it continues the next day, it is likely a sprain or worse.

Whining and crying are obvious signs of pain. If you can't see any obvious injuries or limps, you can run your hands over their body and down their legs. If they whimper or pull back at any point, you have located the sore spot.

Dogs will often hack and cough when they have eaten or breathed in something that doesn't agree with them. Isolated hacking is normal. However, if your dog coughs or hacks routinely during exercise, you could be dealing with a more serious problem. This could be a sign of respiratory infection, heart conditions, and tracheal collapse.

Dogs That Never Stop!

Some dogs just don't stop. High-energy breeds such as border collies, greyhounds, and huskies are usually the guilty parties. They could have a broken leg, but sure enough, you will find them zooming around the house. If you have a dog like this, you are going to need to tighten the reins.

Household changes can make a big difference. While most dogs will stop trying to jump onto the bed when it begins to hurt, high-energy breeds will generally never give up. Start using ramps, and dog stairs in the house, whether your dog thinks they need them or not. If they still enjoy bounding down the stairs after a tumble or two, block the stairs off.

You cannot end their daily exercise routines without chaos ensuing, so it is important to replace activities with ones that are just as rewarding. Make sure to avoid their excitement triggers, or at least change their response to them. For example, if your pup bounds to the bottom of the yard the moment you pick up a ball thrower, you have two choices. You can either stop playing fetch completely, or you can throw the ball short distances with your arm until they realize that they are running too far to catch it. The right choice is easy!

Veterinary Check

Your veterinarian should be your first stop if you are planning out a new exercise routine for your senior pup. They will be able to conduct a full medical examination and give you the green light to exercise. If they feel it is necessary, they may take x-rays to check on the health of your old dog's bones and joints. If they do pick up any medical conditions, they will direct you on which exercises to avoid and which to focus on.

How to Slow Them Down

Whether you're trying to slow down a hyperactive greyhound or trying to get an elderly basset off their butt. The methods below are sure to keep your pup fit, healthy, and injury free.

Find a New Routine

Old dogs like routine. They are already going through changes that they don't quite understand. Introducing any further adjustments can disturb their lifestyle and add to unwanted stress. When switching to a new routine, it is important to taper off physically demanding activities slowly and provide new senior-friendly ones that are just as fun.

Shorter Walks

Walking is a fantastic low-impact, full-body workout. It stretches out muscles, ligaments, and joints, which keeps them flexible and strong. Improved blood flow helps to reduce pain and inflammation, which will provide immense relief from arthritis.

With all these benefits, you can see why your dog should still go on regular walks, even in their older age. However, it is time to go a lot slower. You may notice that they are becoming increasingly sensitive. Their tired little feet will feel the heat of asphalt and the cold of snow more intensely. They will dehydrate faster, and their muscles will tire out quicker.

Keep this in mind when choosing your walking route and avoid walking in extreme weather. Your walks need to be short but consistent, and don't forget to slow down your own pace! If you find your pup feels stiff in the morning, cut down the distance further.

Indoor Exercises

If you find that you are indoors more than out, switch up your games to make them house friendly. If your pup loves to play fetch, move the game indoors. You can purchase soft balls that are designed specifically for older dogs. They don't bounce, which saves your lamps! They are soft, which makes them easy to pick up, and when you throw them, they will travel a shorter distance.

Tug of war is a fun game that you can play indoors. It is a great workout for your dog's neck, shoulders, and jaws. Choose a soft fabric rope that will be kind to your dog's mouth. Make sure you play gently and if your dog starts to get too worked up, pause the game until they become calm.

For small to medium dogs, you can even take a lap around the house! Get creative and adapt your normal routine to suit your new lifestyle.

Swimming and Hydrotherapy

Swimming is a great way to keep your dog in shape. It's a full-body workout, but it is incredibly easy on the muscles and joints. Without your dog's full weight on their legs, their joints can stretch and work without strain.

This doesn't mean that you can just throw your pup into the pool. It's best to get into the pool with them and use a special harness to guide their movements and keep them above water. Inflatable devices can also be used to prevent your dog from drowning if they get too tired.

Hydrotherapy was developed for dogs that have suffered injuries such as broken bones, head trauma, and paralysis. There are plenty of specialized canine rehabilitation centers that offer this service. If you are interested in swimming your dog regularly, it is best to visit one of these centers first and ask them to guide you through it.

Physiotherapy

Physiotherapy is a fun way to improve your dog's physical health while bonding with them. Using the palm of your hand, you can rub down your dog's muscles in gentle, slow strokes. This will improve blood flow, which will loosen up knots and reduce inflammation.

After the massage, you can gently stretch out your dog's legs to loosen up their joints. Avoid stretching them when they are in a standing position, as they can lose balance and fall over! Keep the sessions short and sweet with a ten-minute time limit. If your dog pulls away from you or shows any signs of pain, stop for the day. Massaging and stretching your dog before and after walks can greatly improve their mobility and keep them active.

Combating Boredom

A shorter exercise routine is going to lead to boredom. Keep your dog busy throughout the day to stop any unwanted behaviors and prolonged naps. Mentally stimulating tasks will help to keep your dog's mind working, which will combat dementia and senility.

Stimulating Puzzles

Puzzle feeders are a great way to keep your senior's mind sharp. If you use treats with your puzzles, your dog may gain a lot of weight! Instead, use their daily meals in the puzzles to keep their weight stable. Your dog is likely to get bored if you use the same old puzzles. You can switch things up by putting their food deep inside a snuffle mat.

If your dog needs a bit more exercise, you can play hide and seek. Get them to sit and wait, or put them in another room. Hide their food or treats around the house and let them use their noses to find it. Don't hide too many treats as you may forget where they are and if your dog doesn't find them, you are in for an ant invasion.

New Tricks

Despite what they say, you can definitely teach an old dog new tricks. It may be a little harder for your senior to concentrate, but they are still perfectly capable of learning and enjoying training. Choose tricks and commands that are not too physically taxing. That means, no jumping through hoops of fire.

One of my favorite physical tricks that are light on your dog's knees is dancing. You can train your pup to walk in between and around your legs using hand signals and treats. Put this to a song, and it is a great three-minute exercise for both of you.

Whatever tricks you decide to teach, make sure you do it in moderation. As soon as your pup is getting tired or distracted, it is time to stop.

Play Dates

Your dog will never be too old for friends. Play dates are a great way to spice up your senior dog's routine, and it gives them a chance to just be a dog again. Play dates are mentally stimulating and super exciting. It is physically challenging enough to keep them fit without getting hurt.

This, of course, depends on the playmate. Stick to adult and old dogs that your pup is already familiar with. Introducing them to a young, boisterous puppy that likes to play rough is not going to end well. During the play dates, be mindful of your dog's behavior and if you notice that they get tired or start to feel grumpy, it is time to go home.

Fun In The Sun

Just being in a new place is stimulating enough. Take a trip to the beach or the lake. Have a picnic in the forest or visit a new dog park. You don't need to walk or hike when you get there. Settle down on a blanket and allow your dog to sniff and explore the new world around them.

Chapter 6:

Aging Doesn't Have To Be Scruffy!

Dogs aren't like cats, they don't spend hours grooming themselves with their tongues. Grooming occurs when they partake in everyday activities. As they run, their claws are filed down naturally. Chewing bones and food helps to dislodge any plaque build-up in their teeth. Even just running through bushes or rolling on the grass, is a normal way for your dog to groom their fur.

As your dog ages, their bodies begin to slow down and while they might still enjoy a good roll on the grass, they aren't able to keep up with their usual grooming routine. You may have noticed that your dog suddenly has bad breath, or trouble chewing. When they walk across the wooden floor, they leave behind a trail of scratches! Their once easy-to-brush fur is matted, and you find yourself wiping away gunk from their eyes every day. This is all incredibly uncomfortable and if you don't keep up with regular grooming, it can actually begin to impact their health.

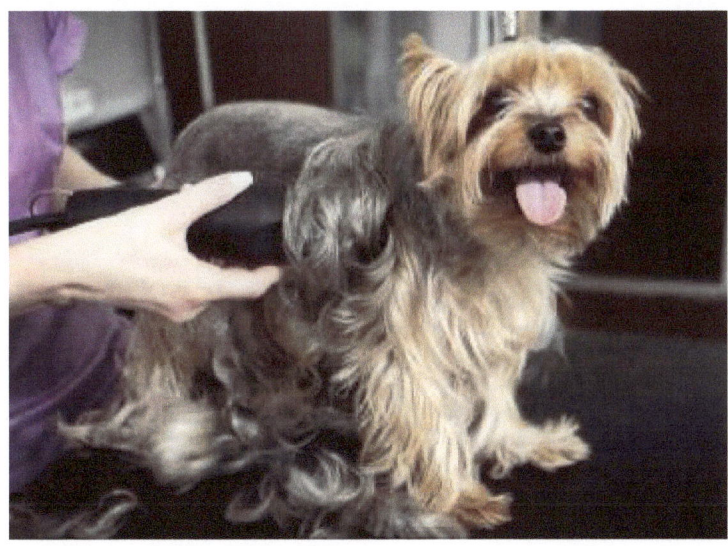

Haircuts and Fur Maintenance

Common Problems

Whether your pup has short and thin fur or long and thick fur, you are likely to encounter some sort of issue as they age. Thankfully, these problems are pretty easy to fix with a regular grooming routine.

Dermatitis

Older dogs become sensitive to chemicals, foods, and plants as they age. These sensitivities can cause mild allergic reactions, which lead to very itchy skin. Dogs suffering from these allergies will lick and chew their skin until it becomes raw. You may notice that they have patches of bare skin and, in severe cases, wounds. While it is best to treat these medically, regular baths with specialized shampoos can soothe the skin and reduce the itch.

Matted Fur

Matted fur is uncomfortable at best, but it can also affect your dog's ability to regulate their body temperature. They use their fur as insulation and if it is matted, the cold will seep in, and they may start to shiver.

Sensitive Areas

Seniors that are prone to potty accidents, will often have matted fur around their sensitive areas. This is due to urine and faces collecting in the fur, which makes it tangle. It looks terrible, smells terrible, and it is extremely uncomfortable for your dog. If left, the bacteria build-up can cause skin and urinary tract infections.

Wounds

Just like people, your dog's skin will begin to thin and lose elasticity, making them more prone to cuts and sores. If your dog has long, thick fur, you may not even notice them until the fur becomes matted around it. Bacteria and dirt will stick to any discharge or blood and can infect the wound.

Grooming

Dogs will generally need to be fully groomed every four to six weeks. This would include a haircut, wash, dry, pedicure, and a face wash. However, these grooming sessions can take up to an hour, depending on the size of your dog and their fur type. Senior dogs can simply not stand that long. Even if they are laying down, the constant noise and rubbing are simply too exhausting.

Instead of one big groom, split it up into shorter, ten minute sessions over a day or even a week.

Regular Brushing

Regular brushing is the best way to keep your dog clean and free of knots. They are much more prone to matting, and you may find you need to brush them daily to keep up.

You will need to ditch the old brushes and invest in gentle ones that have soft bristles. Slicker brushes are great for seniors as they don't snag on tangles or scrape the skin. Small gentle brushes the size of a toothbrush work really well for facial grooming.

To Shave or Not to Shave?

This is quite a debated subject. Older dogs are more susceptible to the cold, so many owners like to keep their coats long. However, old dogs are also more susceptible to matted fur, skin conditions, and infections. Ultimately, the choice is going to depend on what conditions your dog is suffering from and if you can keep up regular grooms to keep their fur healthy.

While a full-body shave may not be the best option for your pup. There are definitely areas of the body that can greatly benefit. Ears, faces, paws, and butts should be regularly maintained, whether it is a full shave or a trim.

For fur in between their paw pads and inside their ears, I suggest using a cordless mini clipper. These are awkward areas to get into, and it is difficult to see where the skin is. The clippers are designed with a safety feature that prevents you from nicking the skin.

Long fur around your dog's face should be trimmed to a reasonable length. This will stop it from poking into their eyes, nose, and mouth and collecting bacteria and gunk. I prefer to use scissors to trim around my dog's eyes and nose.

Shaving or at least trimming your senior's sensitive areas will prevent any urine and feces from becoming matted in the fur. It will also make it much easier to clean them if they have had an accident.

If you want to do a full-body shave, grab yourself a large pair of corded clippers. The large size allows you to do a quicker cut. You can also change the blade, depending on how short you want the fur. Always shave with the grain, not against it.

I like to get my dogs into a comfortable laying down position first. I shave as much area as I can and then give them a short break. They need to stand for their tummy and leg shaves, so I try to get that done as quickly as possible and if needed, I give them another break in between.

Bathing

If you keep up with regular brushes and shaves, then bath time should be a quick affair. Grab your supplies and brush out any knots and matted fur. A mild natural shampoo works well, but you may need to use an antifungal or antibacterial one if your dog has a skin condition.

Using a non-slip mat and keeping them in a seated position will keep them from sliding around the tub. Make sure that the water is at body temperature, you don't want it too hot or cold. Wash them gently and be sure to rinse off all the soap before you take them out.

Don't worry about washing their faces at this point. This can be done later, it is more important to get their bodies dry.

Drying

Always dry your pup after a bath. Even if it is a hot day, you need to dry them! Seniors struggle to regulate their body temperature, and the drastic change from a warm water bath to a cold room will leave them a shivering mess. Use a towel to get the bulk of the water off their fur, but make sure to rub gently so that they don't lose balance.

Thereafter, you should use a hair dryer. Always use it on the lowest possible settings and never focus the dryer on one spot as it can burn their skin. Make sure that their chest, ears, and armpits are completely dry.

Dental Care and Cleanings

Common Dental Problems

Around 80% of dogs will suffer from dental infections at some point in their lives. The pain and discomfort will affect their appetite, and they will begin to lose weight.

Periodontal Disease and Gingivitis

These diseases are caused by a build-up of plaque and bacteria. Senior dogs are more susceptible due to their lowered immune system and change in diet. Dogs that are suffering from gum disease will often have terrible breath, and you may notice frequent bleeding in their mouth.

Grab a flashlight and open their mouths to check for infection. Their gums will be red, swollen, and tender to the touch. If your pup winces when you lift their lips, you are already in for trouble. A build-up of plaque is quite noticeable and can stain the teeth brown if left for long enough. If the infection is not treated, the bacteria can enter the bloodstream and impact vital organs such as the heart, kidney, and liver.

Broken or Filed Teeth

Your dog's teeth will naturally file down with age. There is no reason to be concerned when this happens, and the worst thing that can happen is that your dog won't be able to shred through whole foods.

Broken teeth are common in seniors, as their teeth become brittle after so much wear and tear. This usually occurs when they bite down on something hard or if they sustain an injury. Broken teeth are incredibly painful and will quickly become infected if not treated.

Teeth Cleaning

Brushing your dog's teeth should become part of your weekly grooming routine as they enter their senior years. Preventing gum disease and tooth decay is much easier and cheaper than dealing with infections and tooth extractions.

Chewing and Food

Your dog will naturally clean their teeth when chewing on bones and hard, bulky foods. These are likely no longer options for your senior, but there are some other tricks that can help.

Soft rubber chew toys with bumps and spikes on them work wonders to loosen up any food and plaque that could be trapped in their teeth.

You can also buy dental chews, which are tasty treats that contain ingredients that break down plaque and bacteria.

If your senior dog can still chew kibble, it is worth adding in a few to their meals!

Toothbrushes and Pastes

Doggy toothpaste is not the same as human toothpaste. Most human toothpastes will contain high levels of sodium and xylitol, which can cause serious illness. Pet-friendly toothpastes are completely natural and only contain ingredients that are safe for your pooch to swallow.

While you can technically use a human toothbrush for your dog, you risk them swallowing the bristles if they break. Some brushes are also too hard and can hurt the gums. Dog toothbrushes will usually have soft plastic bristles on the end. You can buy ones that look similar to human ones but are much longer and have a slight curve which allows you to get right to the back of their mouth.

Your other option is a toothbrush that slips over your finger. This makes it a little easier for you to navigate their mouth, but should only be used if you trust them not to nip you!

How To

The hardest part about brushing your dog's teeth is getting them to let you do it. Ideally, you want to train your dog from a young age, but most seniors are pretty good at learning new grooming routines. Start off by getting them used to you touching their mouth. Speak to them gently and give them pats and a couple of treats when they are calm. You can then move on to getting them used to the toothbrush and the taste of the toothpaste. Once they are comfortable and intrigued, you can go in for the clean!

Grab your brush and put a drop of toothpaste on the bristles. Start at the front of your dog's mouth and brush gently in a circular pattern.

Add more toothpaste if needed and slowly work your way to the back of their mouth.

Veterinary Dental Cleanings

Brushing your dog's teeth once a week is a good way to maintain dental health. However, it is still recommended that your dog gets a full dental cleaning at least once a year. During the cleaning, your veterinarian will also be able to take x-rays and check for any decay and broken teeth. If they need to, they will extract any dead teeth.

This process can be a little stressful for owners as your dog will need to be put under anesthetic. Don't worry too much, the veterinary team knows exactly what they are doing! Your dog will undergo a medical examination and at this point, you will need to disclose any strange behavior, medications they may be on, and if they have any allergies to medications. If your veterinarian is happy with their health, they will continue with the cleaning.

Claw Health and Trimmings

There are two parts to a dog's claw. The quick, which supplies blood to the claw, and the end tip and casing known as the shell. The quick is full of nerves, and cutting into it can cause extreme pain and bleeding. This is the fastest way to ensure that your dog never lets you cut their claws ever again.

The quick is a light pink color, which is easy to see if your dog has light-colored claws. If your dog has black claws, you will need to do some guesswork and be cautious not to cut it during trims. If your pup has not had regular trims, the quick is likely to be quite long. However, with regular manicures, it will recede.

Common Problems

There is no way around it, long claws are guaranteed to cause health problems. Senior dogs are more susceptible to these, as their joints and muscles are already taking on a lot of strain.

Broken Claws

Stubbing your toe sucks. Breaking your toenail during that stub warrants the use of every forbidden word in the book. Dogs that have long claws are more likely to get them snagged on furniture, fabric, and paving. While we can treat our broken claws quickly, your dog has to wait for you to notice. Broken claws will often need to be treated by a veterinarian. In severe cases, they may need to surgically remove the entire claw.

Arthritis and Injury

Long claws reduce your dog's traction, which makes it more likely for them to slip and injure themselves, but that's not the worst issue. If the claw hits the ground, it pushes back into the toe and places pressure on the foot and leg.

That pressure can cause tendon injuries, early arthritis, and in severe cases, deformed feet. All of these are incredibly painful, and dogs will typically shift their weight to their hind legs to compensate, which can cause backache.

Claw Clipping

You want your dog's claws to be long enough for them to use, but short enough to avoid any discomfort. If your dog's claws touch the floor when they are standing, they are too long. If you can hear them walking toward you, they are too long!

Before you get started, make sure that you have everything you need. This includes your clipper or grinder, cotton pads, and plenty of treats. I recommend buying a product like Kwik Stop, which helps to stop any bleeding if you accidentally cut the quick.

Clippers and Grinders

There are three types of tools that you can use to cut your dog's claws.

Standard nail clippers work in the same way that human nail clippers do, but they have a curved edge to suit the shape of a dog's claw. You can buy different sizes and strengths to suit your dog breeds.

Guillotine trimmers have a hole at the end of the tool. You put your dog's claw through this hole and then squeeze. This is a great tool for large dogs that have thick claws, as you don't have to squeeze as hard.

Grinders are essentially dremels that have been modified for pooches! You can buy cordless ones that work well for small dogs or larger corded ones that pack more power for thick claws. I love these as you are less likely to cut into the quick of the claw, and you can smooth the edge of the claw. The only downside of using a grinder is the sound it makes.

How To

Get your dog into a comfortable position and hold their paw firmly. You want your thumb on the toe pad and your finger on top. Placing pressure on the pad will push your dog's claw out. You want to clip the tip of the claw straight across. Give your dog a treat before and after every cut to reward them for their good behavior.

If you are using a grinder, you will need to get your dog acclimatized to the sound first. Leave it on and give them a couple of treats. Use it on the tip of a claw and then treat them again. When they are calm, you can grind away! Filing the claws will cause a lot of dust, so be sure to do this in an open area.

The dewclaw is located on the inside of the front leg. Not all dogs have them, but those that do, usually don't use them enough for them to file down naturally. It's important to keep these clipped too as they snag easily.

For indoor pets, it is best to trim the claws every three to four weeks. If your senior still enjoys a stroll, you may be able to push it to five weeks.

When to Worry

If your dog's claws are embedded in their skin, you need professional help. A groomer will have enough experience to file down the claws without causing any further injury. Keep an eye on those paws, though. Open wounds need to be treated and kept clean.

Eyes, Ears, and Nose

Common Problems

Your eyes, ears, and nose are all vital sense organs and any disruption to their normal function can be incredibly frustrating. Without proper grooming, you may find that your dog struggles to see and hear. If left untreated for long periods of time, infections and complete sense loss can occur.

Gunky and Weeping Eyes

Weeping or gunky eyes are not unusual and are not always a cause for concern. Dogs' eyes naturally expel any dust and dirt that has become trapped. You will likely notice this first thing in the morning when they wake up. The discharge should be a normal white to a gray color with a watery consistency.

If the fur around your dog's eye is thick, this discharge may become trapped and collect dirt, which causes tear stains. Again, this is not necessarily a problem as long as there are no other symptoms.

Your dog's eyes should be bright and clear, and the white of the eye should be just that, white! If you notice that the eye has a film over it or the white of the eye is red, this is likely a sign of conjunctivitis. This is a very itchy condition! Dogs that have conjunctivitis will often paw at their eyes and blink excessively.

Ear Infections and Blockages

Dogs that are suffering from ear infections and blockages will typically paw and scratch behind and inside their ears excessively. It can get to the point where they actually scratch their skin open, leaving bare patches and wounds. It can be caused by a dirt build-up, injury, and moisture in the ear that can't dry out.

Dogs that have long fur around the ears are more likely to experience a dirt build-up and infection. It's important to keep the furs around the ear cut short to prevent this. Some dogs are also just gross. They love to roll in anything disgusting and on many occasions, I have had to sit and clean out some nasty substances in and around my dog's ear.

Runny and Dry Noses

Runny and dry noses are not always a cause for concern. Dry noses are commonly a sign of sunburn and, in extreme cases, dehydration. Runny noses are usually caused by mild allergies and any irritants they may have sniffed up. There are a few simple treatments and cleans that you can do at home to provide immediate relief.

Eye Cleaning

It is relatively easy to clean your dog's eyes, and it is one of the grooming activities that most dogs don't seem to mind. You should clean them every time you bathe them, but pups that are prone to eye discharge and tear stains require a wipe down every day or two.

How To

Using a damp cotton cloth, gently wipe your dog's eye. Start in the middle of the eyelid and wipe to the outer or inner edge to push any gunk out. Rinse out the cotton cloth often to ensure that you aren't wiping any gunk back into the eye. If you notice that there is a lot of debris, you can use a saline eye wash to flush it out.

For thick tear stains, you can hold the damp warm cotton cloth over the hair to loosen it. Then brush the debris out with a comb. If the discharge has gone hard, you need to repeat this step throughout the day. Do not tug the fur as it will pull the soft skin around the eye and cause pain.

Once their eyes are clean, you will need to trim the fur around their face. Focus on any longer hairs that may poke into their eyes. Any thick fur under the eyes should also be trimmed to a reasonable length, as these hairs can collect dirt.

When to Worry

If you notice that the discharge has changed to a greeny-yellow color or become thicker, your dog may be suffering from an eye infection. Bloodshot and excessively watery eyes are also symptoms of eye infections and conjunctivitis.

The only thing you can really do is rinse their eyes out with saline solution to remove any debris that may be stuck. This will help relieve the itch. In most cases, conjunctivitis and any other infections will need to be treated with a topical antibiotic ointment, which can be purchased from your veterinarian.

Ear Cleaning

It's best to check your dog's ears after every bath to ensure that they are clean and looking healthy. Most dogs don't require regular deep cleaning, and all you need to do is remove any visible dirt.

How To

After their bath, lift their ears and check for any dirt, parasites, and wounds. If it looks clear, you can dip a cotton pad in mineral oil and gently wipe the outer ear to remove any bits of dirt. Do not use a wet cotton pad that could drip water into the ear canal, as this can cause a yeast infection and earache!

If your dog requires a deeper ear clean, you can purchase a specialized ear wash. Be sure to check the ingredients. Good washes have antibacterial and antifungal properties, which can prevent infections. You don't want products that contain hydrogen peroxide or alcohol, as they are too harsh and will dry out the skin and ear canal.

Hold your dog's ear up and pour the ear wash in until the canal is full. Keep your dog's ear up and gently massage the base to break up any wax or dirt that may be stuck. Let go of the ear and allow your dog to shake it all out. This is the messiest part of the process, so take a few steps back. Once it is all out, use a cotton cloth to wipe away any excess wash and gunk.

Only use cotton wool and cloths to clean the ear and avoid Q Tips as these can push debris further into the ear canal or even puncture the eardrum. Use the first knuckle on your index finger as a guide to how deep you can go into the ear canal. Any further and you risk causing injury.

When to Worry

If your dog experiences pain at any point, stop immediately! They could be struggling with an inner ear infection and further cleaning will be extremely painful. If you spot any blood, inflammation, blockages, or parasites, you should take your pup to your veterinarian for treatment.

Nose Cleaning

A dog's nose is its guide to navigating the world. We know that they should be moist, but what is the reason behind that? The moisture of the nose holds and absorbs scents from their surroundings, which is part of why their sense of smell is so great. When they lick their noses, they taste the scent, which provides them with even more information. Pretty weird, right? This is why keeping their noses clean and functioning is vital.

How To

If your pup has a dry nose, it could be due to something as simple as dirt. Wipe the nose with a warm moist cloth to remove any gunk and wait for an hour to two.

If it doesn't moisten, and you notice the skin is peeling, it could be due to sunburn. You can purchase a specialized sunburn balm that will rehydrate the skin. Remember, dogs lick their noses repeatedly, so you need to ensure that you find a dog-safe balm that can be ingested. This also means that you are going to have to reapply the balm every hour or so.

Runny and blocked noses are a little more difficult to treat, especially if your dog is unruly during grooming. First off, you will need to clean any debris and muck around the nose. You can do this with a warm cloth and a mild soap. If you opt for soap, make sure to rinse it off completely!

Next, clean up around the nose and mouth. If your dog has long hairs that point up into the nostrils, you will need to cut these short. The same goes for any long hairs that trap discharge and dirt underneath. Scissors can be used to cut the hairs, but mini clippers can get the job done quickly without the risk of snipping the skin. This is a great option if your dog is a wiggler.

With the dirt-trapping hairs gone, take your pup into the bathroom and turn the hot tap on in the shower to create steam. The steam will help to loosen up any mucus in the nose. You can also hold a warm cloth at the top of the nose and gently massage it.

This should relieve some irritation and blockage. Your dog's nose is likely to run, so you will need to ensure that you wipe away the discharge often.

When to Worry

Dry noses are also a symptom of dehydration and illness. If you find that their nose is dry for an extended period, it is time to worry.

If you can't get your dog's nose unblocked, and it has started to affect their breathing, you will need to schedule a check-up to find out what is going on! Your veterinarian may use a sinus rinse to clear the nose, which will provide immediate relief. If the discharge is a yellow-green color, or you notice blood in it, your dog may have a respiratory infection.

Chapter 7:

Senior Dog Life Hacks

Adapting to senior life can be tricky. Your dog can no longer do the things they love without feeling discomfort or getting hurt. The loss of these abilities is frustrating and confusing, and they often feel left behind and scared.

While some senior dogs slow down by themselves, others haven't quite figured out that they aren't spring chickens anymore. You have likely already made changes to your environment and lifestyle to accommodate them. However, depending on your dog's personality, not all of these changes will work when put into practice. Adapting these changes slightly can make a significant difference in your dog's quality of life.

If there is something specific you are struggling with, chances are, somebody has already dealt with it and solved it before! Below are some outstanding dog-approved life hacks that I first learned during Sam's senior years.

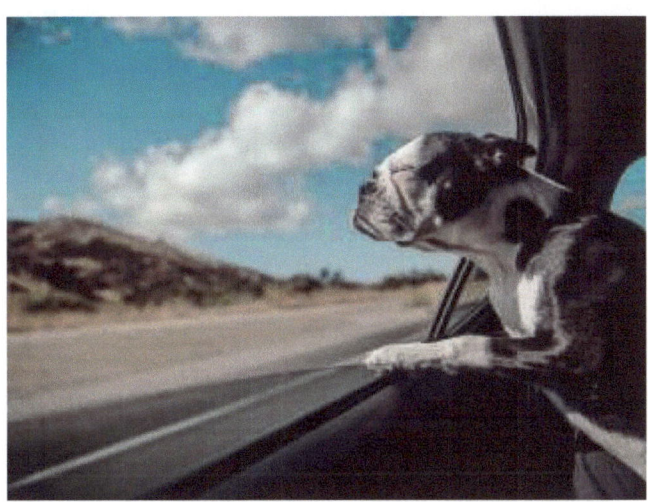

Bumpy Car Rides

If you have a small, senior dog that likes to look out of the window while you drive, then this hack is for you! During the summer months, we would often travel to the lake, which is three hours away. Ordinarily, it was just Sam and I and he would sit in the front seat next to me. One of his favorite things to do was look out the window and enjoy all the new sights, sounds, and smells.

However, as he aged, he began to lose his balance and would frequently fall. If I had to use the brakes, no matter how softly, he would fall against the dash and onto the floor. He would desperately scramble back up onto the seat, scared to miss anything exciting, but the moment I started to drive again, he would slip between the seat and the door!

These once tranquil trips quickly turned into a nightmare. One day, while we were packing up and getting ready to head home, I got an idea! I packed my laundry bag, pillows, and blankets on the floor until it was level with the passenger seat. Every time I had to brake or accelerate, Sam would have a soft space to land if he lost his balance.

As time went on, I noticed that he was only able to stand for a few minutes to look out the window before getting tired. I stacked up the pillows a little higher so that he could lie down comfortably and watch the world go by. The only negative thing about this hack is that I wish I had thought of it sooner.

Wait, Don't Jump!

Elderly dogs, regardless of their size, need to be helped in and out of the car. Even if they look like they can make it, don't let them do it. I once made the mistake of allowing Sam to jump out by himself. The next thing I knew, he was lying on the driveway screaming.

I immediately panicked and picked him up to console him, and he began yelping every time I touched his front leg. We hopped straight back into the car and sped off to the veterinarian for an x-ray.

Thankfully, it was just a sprain and the only treatment needed was love and rest. I wrapped his little leg up with some flexible bandage tape, and he was able to put his weight on it with minimal limping. After a few days, he was back to his normal self.

I got lucky that day, and the injury he sustained could have been much, much worse. Sam was a smaller dog, and it was easy enough to pick him up to put him in and out of the car. For my larger dogs, I use a sling. This helps me to pick them up without breaking my back! Ramps work especially well for giant dogs, and they are easy to move and store.

The Floor is Like Ice!

If you have hardwood floors or tiles, there is no doubt you have watched your dog skid across the room. Sam would bolt down the carpeted stairs and as soon as he hit the wood floor, he would go sliding like a hockey puck and slam into the furniture.

While this was absolutely hilarious to us when he was a young pup, it became dangerous as he aged, and it was only a matter of time before he hurt himself. Even while standing still, his four little paws would slide. It was as if he were standing on ice, and he would constantly shuffle his paws to try to keep his balance.

There is a surprisingly simple fix to this problem. Using a mini clipper, I would remove all the fur I could from in between his paw pads. I would regularly trim his claws to keep them short. This helped tremendously with the sliding.

I Can't Get To Bed

Does your little dog sleep in your bed? Well, then you have probably noticed that they are having trouble mastering the jumps they were once capable of. As they age, their joints become stiff and they develop arthritis. They simply aren't as limber as they once were, and this is unlikely to change.

If they are having to make a second or third attempt to jump onto the bed or sofa, it is time to make a change before they hurt themselves! The good news is, there is an easy fix to the issue. Buy a set (or two, or three) of pet stairs to put next to your bed or sofa. Your furry little friend will now be able to access the snuggles they rightly deserve.

The Stairs Are Too High!

While pet stairs are easy enough to navigate, your senior dog is likely to struggle with taller staircases. These could include porch stairs, deck stairs, and the most troublesome, staircases within the home.

You may have noticed that they struggle to climb the stairs, or they sit and cry, asking for you to help them. If you have deck stairs, your pup will probably choose to potty on the deck rather than use the stairs to access the yard. In the worst-case scenario, they begin to tumble down them, which can cause serious injury.

If you have a small or medium size dog, it is time to start picking them up and carrying them up and down the stairs. For larger dogs, I suggest you build a doggie ramp on shorter staircases, such as porch stairs. If they are struggling up your home stairs, you can use a sling lift to assist them.

If your dog has unsupervised access to your home, I recommend installing a baby gate at the bottom of the stairs to ensure that they can't use the stairs without you. This will reduce the risk of injury and keep your furry friend safe.

I Feel Scared

Living in a multi-dog household, I have had to navigate many personalities, and accommodate my dog's likes and dislikes accordingly. Some of my dogs love the crate, so I have always had one set up in my living room. When not in use, I leave the door open so that they can use it when they please. Sam, on the other hand, hated being closed up in it, which is why it was such a shock to find him curled up in it!

As he aged, his hearing and eyesight deteriorated and his awareness and alertness dwindled. The crate had become a safe haven for him and when he wanted to nap, he was able to curl up inside of it. This sense of security is vital for an aging dog, and it gives them a chance to get some peace and quiet away from the other pets.

If you have other pets, and you don't own a crate, this is a good time to invest in one.

What is Growing on Me?

As Sam aged, he began to develop these little moles all over his body. Some of which grew to the size of a pea! Of course, I was worried, so we went to the veterinarian for a check-up. She explained that they were benign lipomas and there was nothing to worry about. Due to his age, it would be harder for him to go through removing them than it would be to just live with them.

However, they quickly become too gross to handle! They would ooze and bleed, which would then dry in his fur and smell. This made him uncomfortable, so I decided to keep his fur shaved short and bathe him every week to soothe his skin. While he was more comfortable, the cold hit him a lot harder and my other dog began to clean the exposed wound. Other than being disgusting, it also caused Sam more pain as the lipomas were constantly opened.

To solve both problems, I bought Sam an entirely new wardrobe. He had T-shirts for warm days and sweatshirts and sweaters for colder days. These kept him warm and stopped my other dog from licking them. The lipomas were no longer exposed to dirt and bacteria and when they oozed or bled, I could easily change his soiled shirt and treat them.

I Don't Want a Haircut

Sam never really enjoyed being groomed, but it has always been a necessity, especially once the lipomas developed. As he got older, the groomers were no longer able to work with him as he could not stand for long periods of time. It couldn't be that hard to groom him, I thought. So, I set out to purchase a large corded pet clipper and a battery-operated mini one.

They were easy enough to use, but Sam was not having any of it. He refused to stay on the kitchen floor, he would try to bite the clippers and every time he got the chance, he would run away from me. I tried to use a leash, as the groomers did, but every time his heart would race, and he would begin to shake. I couldn't stand it anymore, so I decided to switch it up.

One sunny spring day, I grabbed some towels, training treats, and the clippers. I covered a patio chair with towels so that it was comfortable, and I placed him onto the chair. Sam's favorite thing in the entire world was food, and using treats was the best way to get him to do anything.

I sat in front of him and offered him a treat. I turned the clippers on and gave him another treat. He was still relaxed, so I began to shave him slowly, giving him treats now and then and a bunch of "good boys." I shaved as much of his body as I could while he was laying down and when I got him to stand, I would give him little breaks in between sections.

As we repeated these grooming sessions, he became more and more comfortable, and I was able to use the mini clippers to trim the fur around his ears, snout, and eyes. I still can't believe how much a change of scenery and a bit of comfort changed his mindset!

For larger dogs, you can purchase grooming stands and pillows which can keep them comfortable during the process.

I'm So Cold!

As your dog ages, they begin to have difficulties regulating their body temperature. You may notice that they have started to shiver, even when it feels warm to you! It's important to take this seriously, as they can develop hypothermia if they don't warm up.

Make sure your dog has a sweater for indoors and a warm coat for outdoors. If they sleep at the foot of your bed, get them a warm blanket to snuggle up in. During the winter months, you can place their bed near a heater vent, or fireplace. There are tons of electric heating pads and blankets on the market, and these are a great option for those summer months when you don't want to turn the heater on.

When Did Eating Become Difficult?

As a child, I was taught that dogs only needed to eat once a day. As I got older and adopted my first dog, I realized that dogs are healthier, better behaved, and sleep better at night if they have two meals a day. I realized that Sam wasn't able to stand long enough to actually finish his food. I began feeding him three to four times a day, and noticed an immediate improvement!

Some senior dogs have trouble standing or balancing on tiled or hardwood floors while eating. Placing a rug under their bowls and feeding area can help with their traction, making it easier to stand. Raised food bowls are a great option to solve balancing issues as they reduce the strain on your dog's body.

Their immune system can become compromised, so it is vital to keep their food and water dishes clean!

I Can't Hold it in!

Are you finding yourself cleaning the carpets more often now that your dog has gotten older? Does your furry friend look directly at you while they squat in the middle of your living room? Do you find yourself standing in wet spots when you walk sleepily down the hallway in the morning?

If you do, then you are probably ready to tear your hair out. This is an incredibly frustrating problem to deal with, and you are likely to find yourself angry with your pet, even though you know it is not their fault.

I struggled with this issue for years, and waking up in the middle of the night to let Sam out was not working out well for me. I finally discovered my carpet-saving rescue, doggy diapers! This may sound a little strange, but you can purchase specialized diapers in different sizes for both male and female dogs. Boy diapers are simple wraps that wrap around the belly. Girl diapers look more traditional, and they wrap between their legs and over their rumps.

If you aren't able to frequently change their diapers, you can look at using indoor potty pads. These should only be used on tiled or wooden floors, but placing a towel underneath them can provide extra protection for carpets. It is easy to train your dog to use them, and they work especially well for owners that are at work for most of the day.

I Can't See You!

It's just a matter of time before your furry friend's eyesight begins to deteriorate, and you may notice that their eyes look cloudy or milky. There are a couple of reasons why this may happen, and it is best to get it checked out by your veterinarian. They will be able to find the cause and assess the extent of the eyesight loss. This will give you a better idea of what you are dealing with and what to expect if it were to get worse.

With eyesight loss comes fear, and your dog will have trouble identifying who is coming through the door. To reduce this stress, have your family and friends extend their hands down so that your dog can give them a good sniff. If your dog knows them well and can recognize their voices, you can also ask them to announce themselves before walking in.

This will help keep your dog calm.

I Can't Hear You!

The days of loud, scary thunderstorms are over and the sound of the garbage truck no longer causes a barking frenzy! While this seems like a blessing, there are more cons than pros to hearing loss. During Sam's senior years, I would let him out into the yard to do his business, but when I would call him back, he would stare off into the distance as if he did not hear me.

Calling him for dinner no longer worked, and I found myself shouting his name out, which was not pleasant for anyone. Then one day I smacked my hand against the door and the loud thump caused him to look at me. Eureka!

From then on, I would smack the table or door, or clap my hands until he turned to look at me. I could then motion for him to come, and he happily walked towards me.

Chapter 8:

Life-Changing Products and Tools

I knew that my life would change as Sam reached his senior years, but I never expected how creative I would become! Every time Sam encountered a problem, I found myself heading to the store and grabbing supplies to build some sort of DIY contraption that, I prayed, would help him. Some of it worked, some of it, not so much, but those failures helped me to make something even better. It was a great bonding experience, and I often remember Sam giving me some odd looks when I would whip out the DIY pet sling.

Thankfully, there are a bunch of people out there that are much more creative than I am and have the right tools to build some incredible things. With the pet market booming, there is no end to the remarkable new contraptions that are quickly becoming lifesavers. The great part about the products and tools listed below is that they come in different sizes to suit your dog's breed. Not to mention how much time you will save!

If only these products had been available then, I am confident that Sam would have been a little happier to not have been the test dummy.

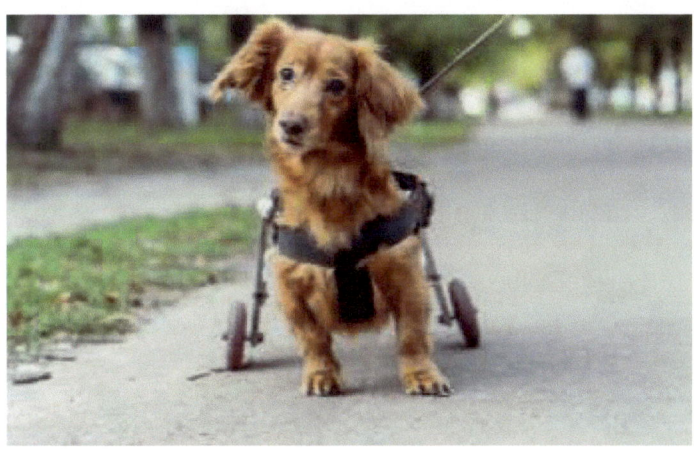

Easy Transport Products

Losing mobility doesn't mean that your dog has to miss out on adventures. There are some fantastic products that ensure your pup enjoys some fun in the sun without any discomfort.

Car Crate

If you find that your dog is struggling to balance and often falls during car rides, it is time to look at getting a car crate. These are a little different from the standard household crates. They are smaller, which restricts your dog's movements, which helps to keep them from falling over. You can purchase them in different materials. Metal mesh crates have a lot of airflow, but they can become uncomfortable if your dog lays against the sides.

Soft mesh crates are much more comfortable and work well for small dogs. Plastic crates are easy to carry and block out the hot sun. Whichever one you prefer, make sure to purchase the right size for your pup!

Car Ramp

Car ramps are an absolute must-have for larger dogs. While jumping up into a car is not ideal, jumping down out of a car is downright dangerous. As your dog lands, they put immense strain on their joints and spinal column, which can cause serious injury. If you have a truck or SUV, it is definitely time to invest in a ramp.

Ramps are foldable, which makes them easy to store and transport. They are coated with non-slip materials, which provide your dog with traction and prevent slipping!

Car Seat Covers

These covers not only protect your seats, but they also protect your dog from falling too! They come in a box shape and clip to the back of your front seats. This prevents your pup from trying to jump into the front seat, and it stops them from falling down onto the floorboard. Seat covers will usually cover the entire back seat, but you can purchase boxed ones for smaller dogs. These follow the same concept but fit snugly on one seat.

If your small dog enjoys looking out the window, you can go one step further and purchase a platformed box seat for them.

Car Seat Extender

These are great for larger dogs that need a little extra room to lay down. It is easy to put them together and pull them apart, which makes it convenient to store them in your trunk. The rectangular shape fits into the floorboards of the back seat, and they have strips that will clip onto your front seats for extra support. This creates a platformed area that essentially extends your back seat into a larger space.

Wagon

Wagons are a great transportation tool for dogs that suffer from mobility issues. They are easy to pull and can be purchased in different sizes to suit all dog breeds. If your dog is recovering from an injury, a wagon is the best way to stick to your normal exercise routine. Even if they are unable to partake in the walk, they can still enjoy the view!

I, personally, enjoy having a wagon with me during longer walks. If my senior pup starts to get tired, they can hop in and take a break without me having to cut the walk early.

Pet Stroller

Pet strollers are the wagon equivalent for small and toy dogs. Strollers do have some advantages over wagons. They can be zipped up, which can prevent your dog from making a run for it. This feature is also ideal for keeping your pup out of the direct sun during those hot days. They are easy to fold, which automatically makes them easy to store and transport. My personal favorite part of having a stroller is being able to toss my water bottle and bag into it.

Bike Trailer

If you and your dog enjoy cycling, it is time to get a bike trailer. These durable mesh trailers run on two or three wheels, depending on size. They clip easily onto the back of your bicycle and are light and balanced, which ensures that you don't fall.

They are designed with mesh tops that can be folded back so that your dog can enjoy the breeze through their very own sunroof. Hardy, rugged ones have been designed for owners and dogs that enjoy camping and forest cycling.

Bike trailers aren't limited to old dog use. They are perfect for any dog that needs a break from an outdoorsy adventure.

Medical Products

Potty Pads

If your pup has been struggling to hold it in, it is time to pick up some indoor potty pads. Disposable pads come in different sizes to cater to all dog breeds, and a lot of them are scented if you are concerned about the smell. They are thick and absorb urine well. However, I recommend using a double layer or purchasing larger ones to avoid any leaks. This is especially helpful for when you are away or asleep, as your pup may need to go more than once.

You can purchase washable potty pads which can be reused. These are a little difficult to use for large dogs but are perfect for small and toy dogs.

If you live in an apartment or your dog is struggling to cope with your porch stairs, you can use a grass potty pad. These are usually made of artificial grass which is placed on top of a tray. It is easy to wash and there is no need to deal with urine smells indoors.

Dog Diapers

Doggy diapers can be used for seniors that have frequent accidents, even while asleep. They come in different sizes and can be purchased for males or females. While the design is different, the structure is identical to baby diapers. This means the cheaper you go, the less effective they are. Mid-range diapers soak in the urine and turn it into gel to avoid any leaks. It is important to remember that doggy diapers are not made for poop, so they cannot be worn all day. Using these in conjunction with potty pads is a great way to avoid accidents.

Slings and Harnesses

While similar to normal harnesses, slings will typically wrap under your dog's belly, close to their hind legs. They are mainly used to assist dogs that are recovering from spinal or limb injuries. However, new slings and harnesses have been developed especially for aging dogs. The sling has a handle that allows you to lift your dog off the floor without breaking your back.

The best part about using slings is that your dog is still able to walk, climb stairs and even perform small jumps. The only difference is that you are keeping the bulk of their weight off the ground, which takes the strain off their joints. Some of the new slings that have been developed can be worn all day, which allows you to assist your pup when they struggle to get out of bed.

Hip Support Braces

If your dog is struggling with hip mobility, you can look into buying support braces. These wrap around the hips and top of the hind legs and then connect to a standard harness. They hold your dog's hips in a secured position, which allows them to walk freely without discomfort.

These can be purchased for dogs of any size, but it is best to get them correctly fitted by a veterinarian or rehabilitation assistant. If they don't fit well, they can cause more harm than good.

Braces should be used to support senior dogs with lower back pain, arthritis or early symptoms of hip dysplasia. If your dog is suffering from a more serious condition, you should consider a doggy wheelchair.

Doggy Wheelchairs

You can buy two types of wheelchairs, one with two rear wheels and one with four. Which one you choose will depend on what kind of support your pup needs. They are generally used for dogs that have suffered from an injury or paralysis. However, they are incredibly helpful for senior dogs with severe arthritis or leg weakness.

They are fully adjustable and can be purchased for dogs of all sizes. No need to cancel that camping trip! You can even change the wheels to suit different types of terrain.

Grooming Support Pillows and Stands

Grooming stands and pillows were developed to keep unruly dogs still during grooming sessions. However, they double up as great support devices for senior dogs. They fit under your dog's belly and keep them in a standing position. The tops are padded to keep your dog comfortable and stop any chaffing. This position makes it easy for you to access all areas of their body, making grooming much, much quicker.

You can purchase them in different sizes, and most are adjustable. For seniors, getting the height right is vital, as this will help keep the bulk of their body weight off their joints! Just be sure to monitor your pup throughout the whole process and give them a break if needed.

Homeopathic Balms

There are tons of fantastic natural balms and ointments that can prevent and treat skin conditions. Doggy sunscreen is a must-have if you have a light-skinned dog. Most of these come in spray form and are quick-drying so that your dog doesn't get a chance to lick it off.

If your pup does end up getting sunburned, you can use a snout soother. This soothes and softens dry, peeling, and burnt noses. Just make sure to check that all the ingredients are edible before applying them.

Your pup's little paw pads will become more sensitive as they age. Walking on snow, hot asphalt, stones, and the rough ground will likely chaff or injure them. You can buy a specialized paw wax that can be used before and after walks. These generally contain antibacterial and antifungal elements. This means the wax will soothe the skin while protecting it from infections.

Tools For A Comfortable Home

Getting old is uncomfortable enough. Adding flat, uncomfortable beds, slippery floors, and couches that are too high to jump on makes getting old an absolute misery. Keep your dog comfortable and cozy with these fantastic products.

Crate

Crates and indoor kennels are great comfort tools for senior dogs. You don't have to purchase the conventional metal one. In fact, using a wooden enclosed one is sometimes better. These crates help to muffle noise and block out light. It also keeps your dog safe from other household pets that enjoy pushing their muzzles through the metal to get a quick sniff.

Orthopedic Beds

If you have a large and heavy dog, these are VITAL. Most dog beds start off nice and fluffy, but after a few washes they are flat, and your dog ends up sleeping on the hard floor. Orthopedic beds have thick memory foam mattresses that keep their shape and keep your dog's hips intact. You can buy ones that lay flat on the floor or elevated ones. Elevated ones are great as they add a little extra protection from the cold floor in winter.

When buying a bed, it is important to make sure that it is actually big enough for your dog. You don't want their heads falling off the side. If your pup does enjoy stretching out, you can purchase ones that have L or U-shaped pillows, which will stop them from rolling off.

Heated Dog Pads

Heat pads are a great source of warmth and comfort for pets of any age. Senior dogs that struggle to keep warm or suffer from stiff joints and arthritis benefit the most from these. The heat is soothing and promotes blood flow, which eases digestive pain and reduces inflammation. You can purchase them in different sizes to suit your breed, and they fit snugly under your dog's bed or blanket.

They usually have three different settings which allow you to adjust the temperature, which means you can use it in warm weather too!

Pet Stairs and Ramps

We already know that pet stairs are great. They are light and easy to set up next to your bed or couch. Your pup can now get up and down without taking any strain on their joints. Mini ramps are very useful, especially if you have a toy dog that may struggle with the pet stairs. You can purchase the ramps in different sizes and heights, which allows you to use them on short staircases and porch stairs.

It's important to not go for the cheaper options if you are buying a ramp for long-term or outdoor use. You want one that is covered with non-slip materials to provide traction for your pup.

Traction Rugs and Mats

Using textured rugs and mats is a fantastic and cheap way to stop your dog from ice skating over hardwood and tiled floors. You don't even need to purchase expensive ones, yoga mats work just as well. As an added bonus, these mats can be used to create pathways through the house to help blind dogs navigate their surroundings.

Raised Dog Bowls

You can purchase raised bowls and stands at different heights to accommodate all sized dogs. Some of them are even adjustable. Lifting food and water bowls off the floor can help alleviate neck and joint strain, as your pet won't need to stay in a bent over position to eat. Simply getting your dog out of that hunched position will promote overall digestive health. Combining these bowls with traction mats is ideal for dogs that are prone to slipping on the floor or losing their balance.

Dog Clothes and Shoes

Fashion and function! By now, you know how important it is to get your dog a warm sweater for those cold days, but there are so many more accessories that will change your senior's life. Waterproof coats are the perfect accessory to keep your dog dry, and you will be able to continue your exercise routine while it is raining. Booties are great for keeping your dog's paws warm during snowy days, and you can purchase light ones that protect their paws from cold floors.

You can now buy upgraded dog shoes that come with non-slip pads underneath. These prevent your dog from slipping across smooth floors and protect their paws on hot asphalt.

If your dog doesn't like wearing booties, you can buy toe grips. Yes, that is a thing! These little rubberized grips fit over your dog's claws. While the grips won't be able to support your dog's ankles, they do help with traction.

Chapter 9:

Knowing When To Say Goodbye

Honestly, this is the absolute worst part of owning a dog. The heartbreak and pain you experience are enough to make you give up on the idea of ever adopting another one. We sadly only get a limited amount of time to spend with our dogs and, unfortunately, we inevitably need to say goodbye. Saying goodbye is not easy, and it is easy for us to get wrapped up in veterinarian visits and treatments to find any way possible to extend their lives for just a few more years. However, we need to remember that this is not just our lives, it is theirs too and when it is time for them to go, we have to let them go. Your duty as an owner is to provide them with the best possible life you can, and this includes a peaceful death.

As we have discussed already, each breed has an estimated lifespan, and some of you may have to say goodbye sooner than others. However, this is just that, an estimate. Each pup is different, and you will need to understand their medical condition and personalities to understand the signs and symptoms.

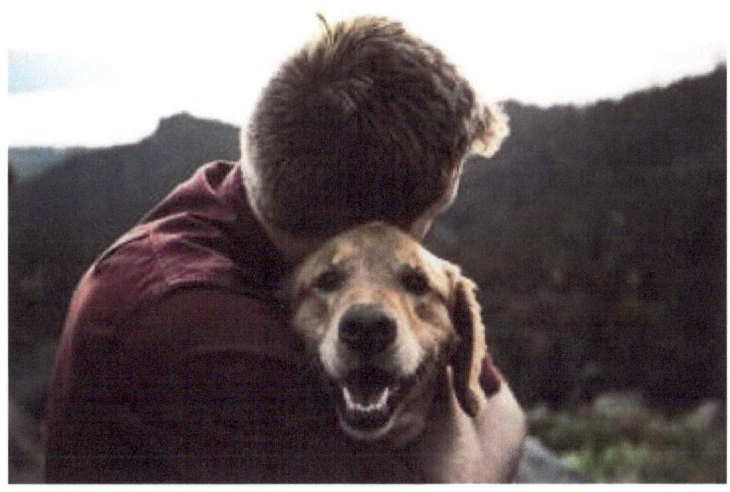

Signs Your Dog May be Ready to Pass

Just because your dog is displaying these symptoms, does not mean that they are days from passing. Your pup could have weeks or months left. Don't let the panic take over! These symptoms are common for a variety of illnesses, and they can be difficult to differentiate. However, if your dog is very old and these symptoms seem to have no cause, you need to get prepared to say your goodbyes.

Appetite

A loss of appetite is a common symptom of stress, illness, and underlying medical conditions. However, through all this, it is likely that your pup will still try to stomach their favorite treats. More often than not, dogs that are ready to pass will completely lose their appetite, including a refusal to eat their favorite foods. This could be accompanied by a refusal to drink water as well.

Lethargy and Disinterest

As we now know, lethargy could be a symptom of several medical conditions. However, when this becomes extreme and there are no medical reasons behind why, you need to prepare yourself. Your dog will likely sleep for long periods of the day, battling to get up and refusing to play or exercise.

Attention-Seeking or Emotional Detachment

Depending on your dog, they will react in one of two ways. A normally loving and cuddly dog may begin to detach itself from you completely. At the same time, a usually independent dog may begin to seek constant attention and comfort. Both are completely normal, and this is just a way for your dog to cope with the inevitable. While emotional detachment is devastating, it is important to remember that this is about your dog, not you. You should provide them with a safe haven and give them their space when they ask for it.

Confusion and Lack of Coordination

Aging can take its toll on the muscles and mind. As the muscles deteriorate and arthritis kicks in, your dog may lose their ability to coordinate their bodies. They may walk into furniture, wobble while they walk, or fall for no reason. This can cause confusion and frustration. Their minds will also deteriorate over time, and they may forget what they were doing, and where they are and even lose their sense of direction.

To keep your dog calm and comfortable, you should reduce the need for them to walk long distances to access food, water, and potty areas. Move their bowls and potty pads into the room where they sleep. Make sure to monitor and assist them if need be when they go outdoors.

Dull Eyes

In the end, there is something distinctly different about your dog's eyes. Almost as if the sparkle that was once there is gone. It's a difficult symptom to describe, but it is unforgettable when you see it. I like to believe that at this point, they had already begun their trot across the rainbow bridge, but decided to turn around and hang on just a little longer to spend those last minutes with you.

Consult Your Veterinarian

There are symptoms that you can manage at home, and there are some that need medical attention. If you notice that your dog is experiencing any of the following signs, seek guidance from your veterinarian.

Illness

Very old dogs are fragile and with their lowered immune system, they are often unable to fight even the simplest of illnesses anymore. Medical conditions are also likely to get much worse at this point. Treating the symptoms will provide your dog with comfort, but if you think that your dog is suffering in any way, get them the help that they require.

Pain

Pain is the worst symptom you could hope for. There is nothing more distressing than watching your dog suffer. If they are experiencing pain, crying out, or whimpering, you will need to take them for a check-up. Depending on the severity, your veterinarian will give you pain medication which will make them more comfortable. Worst-case scenario, your veterinarian may speak to you about euthanasia.

Breathing Difficulties

A change in breathing is a completely natural sign that your dog may be nearing their last hours of life. If your pup is comfortable and happy, let them be. Put a light blanket over their body to keep them warm and be sure to stay by their side. However, if you can see that they are in pain, gasping, or becoming increasingly panicked, call your veterinarian straight away.

Total Incontinence

Total incontinence occurs when their muscles have become so weak that they are unable to hold it in for minutes at a time. This could also mean that a number of their organs are failing. This is a scary thought, but it is not necessarily painful. Regardless, it can become uncomfortable and even embarrassing for your dog. If they are hiding from you and whimpering when it happens, speak to your veterinarian.

Saying Goodbye

Saying goodbye is overwhelming at best. You will likely be full of strong emotions. Sadness, love, guilt, and even anger can take over. Regardless of how you feel, you will need to remain calm. Speak to them, stroke them gently, and display only love. Dogs can pick up on emotions and body language quickly, and if you are in distress, they may mimic your feelings or try to respond to them.

Getting Them Comfortable At Home

Try to continue your normal daily routines. This will depend heavily on your dog's health, of course. Long walks may not be possible anymore, but keeping up feeding, playing and cuddling routines is still important. A sudden and drastic change in routine and daily activities can lead your dog to feel confused and isolated.

Limit their pain. Use pain management medication and homeopathic remedies to reduce pain and inflammation. This will greatly improve their quality of life and allow them to enjoy their last few weeks. Stronger medications may be needed toward the end.

A warm, comfortable, and quiet spot for them to relax is the top priority. You do not want your dog to suffer in any way. Eliminate the cold, the pain, and the noise, and you will see an immediate improvement in their behavior.

Sometimes this is unavoidable, but if you can, don't let your dog go alone. Being able to have that last cuddle is a great comfort for them, and they can go with ease. This is also a critical part of the grieving process for you. If you are unable to be home at all times, ask a friend or family member to dog-sit them for you. It is not the same as being there yourself, but at least you can rest assured that they weren't alone and received love until the very end.

Medical Intervention

Medical intervention is generally only needed for dogs that have been struggling with chronic conditions and illnesses. This is the most difficult way to say goodbye, and many owners find themselves riddled with guilt afterward. Your responsibility has always been to your dog, keeping them healthy, happy, and full of love. You will need to take this into account for their death as well. A quick, peaceful goodbye is better than your dog spending their last days in pain and discomfort.

What Is Euthanasia?

Your veterinarian will not take the decision to euthanize lightly, and they will ensure that there is nothing more that they can do before they recommend it. If the decision is final, your dog will be taken to a quiet room and made comfortable. You will be given time to say your goodbyes, and you will have the option of being with your dog during the procedure.

Your veterinarian will then inject your dog with an overdose of anesthetic. This is completely painless, and your dog will fall asleep before the injection is even finished. They will then pass peacefully within a matter of minutes.

Should I Stay With My Dog?

A veterinary practice is a strange and sometimes scary place. Being in this environment can be quite distressing to your dog, and they aren't able to understand what is happening or why they are there. During any other veterinary visit, you are there to comfort them and hold their paw during the check-ups. Suddenly being alone in there is just too confusing for them.

While the veterinarian and assistants are well-trained and will treat your dog with nothing but love and empathy, it is not quite the same. This will be the last time you can hold them, comfort them, and assure them that they were completely and utterly adored. What more could a dog ask for?

While I always recommend that you stay with your dog, it is completely understandable if you are unable to. If this is something that you know you just can't cope with, it is still important to say your goodbyes before they go. You don't want your dog to go alone and be confused, especially if you were distressed during your final goodbye. Ask a friend or family member that your dog knows and loves to take your place during the procedure.

In some cases, your veterinarian will actually be able to come to your house. This is ideal as your dog can pass in a comfortable space they know and love.

Choosing a Resting Place

Choosing the right resting place for your companion is a critical part of the grieving process. A few years ago, burial was generally considered the only option. It is a great way to say your final goodbyes and have a memorial service. This also provides closure for family members that were not with your pup when they passed. However, if you do not own your property or intend to move to a new city or country, this option is definitely not for you.

If your pup has been put to sleep, you may not be able to take them home to bury them. Cremation is a great option in this case and is often the preferred one overall. This is done by a specialized pet crematorium which will offer a range of memorabilia. Ornate urns are a great option if you want to keep your dog close. Or, opt for a simple box if you intend to spread or bury your pup's ashes. Your veterinarian or the crematorium can even take a paw and nose prints for you. These can be set in stone or printed on paper.

Chapter 10:

Coping With Loss

Each one of us is different. We all process loss in different ways. For some, it may only take a few days to come to grips with the loss of a beloved pet. For others, it can take years. This doesn't make us any stronger or weaker than one another, and it is important to never doubt yourself through this trying period. The loss of a pet is hard enough, you don't need to worsen it for yourself.

Our pets give us a sense of purpose. On our darkest days, they give us a reason to get out of bed. They are a continuous reminder of how beautiful life can be. Yes, they can be a little annoying every so often. You may trip over them or want to scream when you are cleaning up the third pee puddle of the day. Yet, the moment they are gone, you find yourself missing the little things you didn't even realize they did.

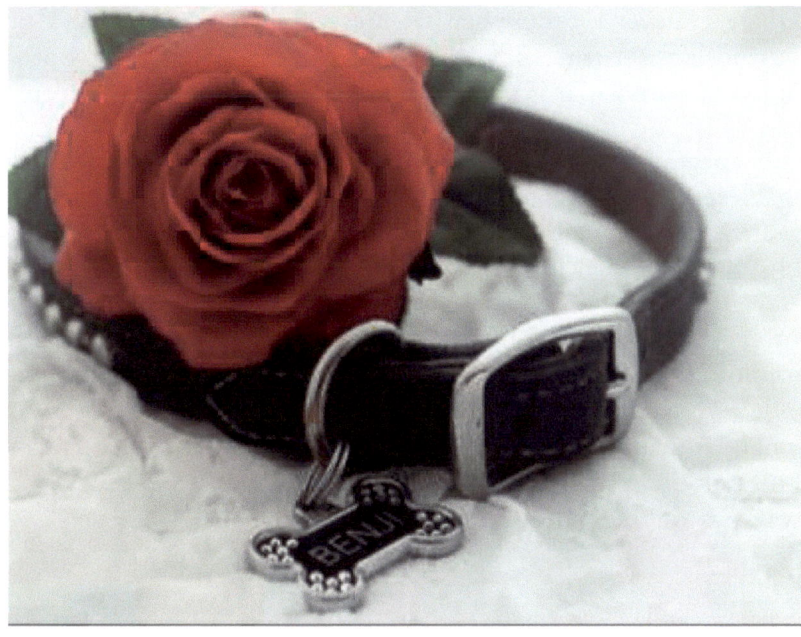

It's Okay To Cry!

Experiencing any kind of loss is overwhelming, yet the loss of a pet hits differently. You are allowed to cry. You are allowed to scream! Don't feel ashamed of your feelings, and never try to bottle them up and forget them. It is so important to accept these emotions, and expressing them can relieve some of the pain you are feeling. Grieving is a long, exhausting, and difficult process and is often harder than being with your dog when they pass. Finding a strong, empathic support system is the only way to get through it.

Be Kind to Yourself

Don't pressure yourself into moving on. There is no allotted time for grief, and the idea that you "should just get over it" is more damaging than mourning for a bit longer. Our pets provide us with so much more love and support than we realize. We set up routines in our lives to care for them and spend time with them. We come home to their excitement each day. Their permanent presence in our home means that there is never a time when we are actually alone. Losing a pet is not just losing a partner. It's losing their love, support, and your daily routine, and purpose. It is no surprise that it is so difficult to accept it.

The unexpected death of a pet can be particularly hard. The guilt of not being there when it happened and feeling as though you could have prevented it can be overwhelming. The constant "what ifs" are not healthy, but as hard as it is, you need to let go of that guilt.

If you feel this way, you shouldn't try to take it on alone. If you have the opportunity to, speak to your veterinarian. They will be able to provide you with insight into what could and couldn't have been done. Which is sometimes all you need to have some closure. Having a healthy support system in which you can express your feelings of guilt without fear of judgment is vital.

Mourn Together

If you have a family or a partner, it is important to remember that they are grieving too. Children are especially affected by the loss of the pet, as most are unable to fully comprehend the concept of death. Take the time to talk it through with them and show them that it is okay to feel sad and express their emotions. Share your favorite stories and remember all the good times you had together. Sometimes, being the support system for others can help you to mourn too.

Believe it or not, dogs can mourn too. Their best friend has disappeared, and they don't understand why. Grieving dogs will often become less active, and you may find that they wander around the house whining or whimpering. This can be worsened as they pick up on what you are feeling. Take the opportunity to mourn together. Spend time together, give them love and attention, and partake in fun activities that will make you both smile.

Join a Support Group

When you grieve, it is only natural to reach out to somebody in hopes of receiving compassion and support. However, some people have never owned a dog, and they have absolutely no idea how the loss of one can impact you. You are unlikely going to get the support that you need from them and in some cases, you may actually feel worse. This isn't their fault. They aren't trying to deliberately hurt you, they just genuinely don't understand how it feels. Support groups may be a much better option for you if you don't have any close friends or family that understand what you are going through.

Joining a group doesn't necessarily mean you have to meet in person, which, let's face it, can be quite scary. Online support groups are a great way to meet people who are going through or have gone through the same loss. These platforms allow people to express their sadness, guilt, and anger without embarrassment or shame. Being able to read about other people's experiences and how they have coped with loss is a great way to get some perspective on your situation and learn new methods of how to cope with loss.

Moving On

You are not betraying your dog by moving on. Don't ever feel guilty about it. The thought of forgetting about them completely is terrifying, but I can assure you that is simply not possible. Dogs have such a big impact on us and while we may forget small details here and there, we can never ever forget their presence. There are tons of ways to document the times you spent together and if you ever feel like their memory is slipping, you can go back and remind yourself.

Memorials

Funerals are a wonderful way to get closure. Once your dog has passed, you will likely realize that there is so much more that you wanted to say or do for them, but just never had the chance. This allows you to say your final goodbyes and let them know how much you loved them. This closure is not just for you. Friends, family members, and especially children that were close to your dog will have the opportunity to say goodbye as well.

Being able to share this moment with the people you love is so important. Each of you should share your favorite story, remembering the best and funniest times you had together. Prepare for laughs and tears.

Create a memorial box to bury with your pet. You can include their favorite toys, collar, and blankets. Writing out your feelings and your most inner thoughts that you may not want to express in front of others can be healing. You can bury your letter with your box.

Mark their burial spot so that you will always be able to come back to it when you are feeling down and want to talk to them. You can do this with a cross or a stone, but I really love to plant flowers or a beautiful tree. If you and your dog had a favorite spot at the doggy park, consider donating a bench with a plaque to remember them.

Scrap Books

Scraps books are another great way to keep your dog close to you at all times. Put in their photos, especially ones of the two of you together. Under each photo, write down a story or a letter to them to ensure the memory lasts a lifetime. You can tape in a piece of their favorite blanket or a scrap of their favorite plush toy as well.

Make sure that you take photos before it is too late! If you don't have any, you can hire a professional photographer and have a doggy photoshoot.

Create a New Routine

This is non-negotiable. You likely have a bunch of extra time on your hands and if you aren't using it properly, you can fall into a deep pit of depression. Find a way to fill this void! Regular exercise is a great way to burn off excess energy and frustration. We have just learned how beneficial it is for the mind, so do not give it up. Meditative and calming routines such as yoga classes can help to increase your mental well-being. Visiting friends and keeping social will bring back some joy in your life. Don't feel guilty about laughing.

Give Back

If you feel that you are ready to be around dogs again, I suggest volunteering at an animal shelter. It may be sad at first, but these are dogs that are desperate for love, attention, and stability. The work you will do there is incredibly important, and you can honor your dog's memory by helping them.

Who knows, you may even meet a pup that needs you as much as you need them.

Sometimes It's Better to Forget

We all grieve in different ways and for some of us, the grief is simply too overwhelming. Being around your dog's things, seeing photographs, meeting other pets, or just hearing their names can send you into hysterics. In times like this, it may be best to forget. It is not possible to forget them completely, but clearing out your home of their memory may help. Donate their things to an animal shelter that would be able to put them to good use. I suggest that you box and store your photographs of them, just in case you want to revisit your time together at a later stage.

It's best to avoid other dogs at this point, but you won't need to do this forever! Most importantly, don't feel guilty. If this is how you are able to cope with loss, then put yourself first and do it.

Adopting a New Dog

Most people that have never owned dogs before will tell you to just get another one. This is not something that should be rushed! Bringing a new dog into a turbulent household is not healthy. You need to make sure that you are in an emotionally stable state before you make this decision. You cannot rely on a dog to fix you.

Replacing a dog is also just not possible. Each pup is so unique and their personalities and traits are wildly different. Trying to replace your dog can lead you to resent your new one when they don't behave the same way. You need to adjust your expectations and be prepared to invite a new, special, and unique animal into your life.

However, that being said, you should not close yourself off from the idea of adopting a new dog. Once you are ready and in the right headspace, your new pup can help you to get back on track. Volunteering at an animal shelter is a great way to test how you feel and if you are actually ready to take this new step. It is also the best way to bond with new dogs, learn their personalities, and find out if you are compatible. Love cannot be forced, and the two of you need to choose each other.

Conclusion

I know that we have ended on a sad note, but it is time to wipe away those tears and focus on the now. Your dog may be in their senior years, but you still have plenty of time left with them. If you put some of these methods into practice, you will likely end up with more time than expected.

Hopefully, at this point, you are feeling a bit calmer and more confident in your parenting skills. You now know how to groom your dog at home, adjust their diets to provide them with tons of energy, and continue a healthy slow exercise routine to keep them fit. If you have been concerned about your dogs' health, I hope that these medical chapters have given you the power to identify their illnesses and seek treatment where necessary. Never forget that prevention is the best form of cure, and your vigilance can save your dog's life.

Caring for your senior dog correctly will not only improve their quality of life but yours too. By letting go of that stress and anxiety, you have opened up space for love and joy. Which is all your dog really wants for you! This kind of energy is healing within itself, and the happier you are, the happier your dog will be.

While things will definitely improve, let's not pretend that there won't be difficult times. There will be ups and downs and laughs and tears. Depending on your dog's condition, you may not be able to do it all alone. Find a support system and seek guidance from your veterinarian and rehabilitation assistants. Use the platforms given to you to further your knowledge and better understand what your dog is going through. Social media support groups are a fantastic place to learn new techniques and life hacks and chat with people who are dealing with similar issues as you. You will find that even these dark days will pass. Stay positive, keep smiling, and enjoy every moment that you have left.

Dogs are such a beautiful gift and while we may become frustrated at times, the love, and joy they bring into our lives are insurmountable.

We are given such a short time together, and it is our responsibility to ensure that their lives are completely fulfilled.

Incorporate all the things that your dog loves to do! If they want to sleep on your bed, let them. If you have never celebrated their birthday, bake them a dog-friendly cake. Have you always wanted to visit that special lake with them? If they are well enough, make the trip. It's time to stop focusing on the destination, and start enjoying the journey.

If you have enjoyed this book, please leave a review on Amazon!

Other Publications:

Adult Dog Training Through Positive Reinforcement: Learn the Essential Skills Needed to Shape an Obedient and Well-behaved Dog

About The Author

I can't remember a time in my life when I was not completely obsessed with dogs! Especially the ones that nobody else wants. Growing up, I had to constantly resist the urge to bring home every stray puppy I saw, and each time, my heart broke a little more. When the opportunity finally arose for me to provide one of these lost souls with the perfect home, I drove straight to the shelter.

However, I soon found myself overwhelmed by all the problems that come with rescuing a dog, so I set out to learn the best way to train and heal my new soulmate. Inspired by my favorite behaviorists and dog trainers, I decided to follow in their footsteps and help as many people and pups as possible.

For the last 30 years, I have dedicated my time to studying different training techniques—the good, the bad, and the ugly—and I came to learn exactly which ones produced the results I wanted. The end goal is never just a trained dog. The goal is a well-adjusted, healthy, and happy dog.

I soon learned that training them was easy, but losing them is hard. When my Gizmo slipped into his senior years, my world was turned upside down. I was so focused on the present that I hadn't put any thought into the future. In those last years, our roles were reversed. He became the trainer, and I, the trainee. The lessons I learned from him have stayed with me forever and prepared me for the inevitable love and loss I would experience again and again.

My books are compiled of tried and true techniques, life lessons, and healthy coping mechanisms that have personally helped me to work with and love my dogs. I am confident that I can provide them the best life from puppy to senior that they deserve and by the time you finish reading this, you will be too.

—Hope Chambers

References

Abraham, M. (n.d.). *Senior dogs | Dog health*. The Kennel Club. https://www.thekennelclub.org.uk/health-and-dog-care/health/health-and-care/a-z-of-health-and-care-issues/senior-dogs/

Advanced Care Veterinary Hospital. (2021, February 2). *Why is it Important to Trim Your Pet's Nails?* Advanced Care Veterinary Hospital. https://advancedpetvet.com/2021/02/02/why-is-it-important-to-trim-your-pets-nails/#:~:text=However%2C%20long%20nails%20create%20potential

AKC Staff. (2015, March 23). *How to Clean Dogs Ears & Eyes*. American Kennel Club. https://www.akc.org/expert-advice/health/eyes-and-ears-of-good-grooming/#:~:text=Healthy%20eyes%20are%20bright%20and

AKC Staff. (2019, November 20). *Your Dog's Age In Human Years: A Conversion Chart*. American Kennel Club. https://www.akc.org/expert-advice/health/how-to-calculate-dog-years-to-human-years/

AKC Staff. (2022a, May 3). *Nutrition and Supplement Tips for Senior Dogs*. American Kennel Club. https://www.akc.org/expert-advice/nutrition/nutrition-and-supplements-for-senior-dogs/

AKC Staff. (2022b, December 13). *A Survival Guide for Dog Diarrhea*. American Kennel Club. https://www.akc.org/expert-advice/health/doggie-diarrhea/#:~:text=Withholding%20food%20for%2012%20to

Alusin, M. (2017, July 4). *5 signs it's time to say goodbye to your dog*. Dog's Best Life. https://dogsbestlife.com/dog-health/5-signs-its-time-to-say-goodbye-to-your-dog/?cn-reloaded=1

Amatenstein, S. (2021, December 14). *How to Cope with The Loss of A Pet*. Psycom. https://www.psycom.net/loss-of-a-pet

America Holistic Veterinary Medical Association. (n.d.). *What is Holistic Veterinary Medicine?* American Holistic Veterinary Medical Association. https://www.ahvma.org/what-is-holistic-veterinary-medicine/

Anastasio, A. (2019, August 6). *Grieving a Pet: How to Cope With the Loss of a Dog*. American Kennel Club. https://www.akc.org/expert-advice/lifestyle/grieving-a-pet/

Animal Hospital of Clemmons. (n.d.). *What can I give my dog for a urinary tract infection?* Animal Hospital of Clemmons. https://www.animalhospitalofclemmons.com/site/veterinary-pet-care-blog/2020/12/18/urinary-tract-infection-in-dogs

Arford, K. (2021, September 1). *Dog First-Aid Kit Essentials: What To Include For Injuries And Emergencies*. American Kennel Club. https://www.akc.org/expert-advice/health/dog-first-aid-kit-essentials/

ASPCA. (2015). *Common Dog Diseases*. ASPCA. https://www.aspca.org/pet-care/dog-care/common-dog-diseases

Australian Veterinary Association. (2019, October 9). *What to do if your pet vomits or has diarrhoea*. Vet Voice. https://www.vetvoice.com.au/articles/what-to-do-if-your-pet-vomits-or-has-diarrhoea/

Bates, A. (2021, March 30). *The Consequences of Dog Inbreeding: Problems & Risks*. Pet Keen. https://petkeen.com/dog-inbreeding-consequences/

Bauhaus, J. M. (2021, August 19). *How to Clean Dog Ears*. Hill's Pet Nutrition. https://www.hillspet.com/dog-care/routine-care/how-to-clean-dog-ears#:~:text=Use%20a%20cotton%20ball%20or

Bednarik, K. (2018, July 9). *The 5 Most Common Chronic Conditions in Cats and Dogs.* Embrace Pet Insurance. https://www.embracepetinsurance.com/waterbowl/article/common-chronic-conditions-in-cats-and-dogs

Bell, J. S. (2017, September 25). Ten Most Common Hereditary Diseases in Dogs. *World Small Animal Veterinary Association Congress Proceedings, 2017.* https://www.vin.com/doc/?id=8506247

Blue Buffalo. (n.d.). *Gently Guide Your Dog through His Golden Years.* Blue Buffalo. https://bluebuffalo.com/articles/dog/gently-guide-your-dog-through-his-golden-years/

Blue Cross. (n.d.). *Time to say goodbye to your dog.* Blue Cross. https://www.bluecross.org.uk/advice/dog/time-to-say-goodbye-to-your-dog#:~:text=Persistent%20and%20incurable%20inability%20to

Bovsun, M. (2020, December 21). *Dog Constipation: Home Remedies and When to Call the Vet.* American Kennel Club. https://www.akc.org/expert-advice/health/dog-constipation/

Bubbly Paws. (2022, May 31). *Is Grooming Safe for Senior Dogs With Health Conditions?* Bubbly Paws. https://www.bubblypaws.com/barkblog/is-grooming-safe-for-senior-dogs-with-health-conditions#:~:text=With%20senior%20dogs%2C%20it%20is

Buddy Blog. (2019, July 18). *How much exercise should an old dog get?* Buddy Rest. https://buddyrest.com/blogs/buddyblog/how-much-exercise-should-an-old-dog-get

Burke, A. (2021, June 21). *Dog Coughing: Causes and Treatment Options.* American Kennel Club. https://www.akc.org/expert-advice/health/dog-coughing-causes-treatment/

Buzby, J. (2015, August 16). *9 Helpful Products for Aging Dogs.* The Grey Muzzle Organization. https://www.greymuzzle.org/grey-matters/health-and-well-being-common-health-issues-care-mobility/9-helpful-products-aging-dogs

Chewy Editorial. (2015, March 30). *Dog Grooming Tips For Senior Dogs*. BeChewy. https://be.chewy.com/dog-grooming-tips-for-senior-dogs/

Chewy Editorial. (2018, July 2). *5 Common Congenital Dog Diseases*. BeChewy. https://be.chewy.com/5-common-genetic-diseases-of-dogs/

CitiVet. (n.d.). *Your Senior Dog*. CitiVet. https://citivetgardens.co.za/dog-old-age/#:~:text=Besides%20the%20usual%20complete%20physical

Clancy, M. (2020, March 31). *13 Essential Items To Have In Your Dog's First-Aid Kit*. Dogtime. https://dogtime.com/dog-health/general/21573-things-in-dog-first-aid-kit

Clark, M. (2021a, April 9). *Gold Souls, Gray Faces: 6 Indoor Exercises For Senior Dogs*. DogTime. https://dogtime.com/dog-health/fitness/62279-indoor-exercises-senior-dogs

Clark, M. (2021b, August 5). *Gold Souls, Gray Faces: 6 Tips For Cleaning Your Senior Dog's Teeth*. DogTime. https://dogtime.com/dog-health/dog-dental-care/64355-cleaning-senior-dogs-teeth#4

Cohen, M. A. (2016, December 4). *The 6 Most Common Genetic Disorders in Dogs*. PetMD. https://www.petmd.com/dog/slideshows/6-most-common-genetic-disorders-dogs

Coile, C. (2020, February 26). *Eating Well Into Old Age: Health And Nutritional Needs For Senior Dogs*. American Kennel Club. https://www.akc.org/expert-advice/nutrition/nutritional-needs-for-senior-dogs/

Cooper, S. (2021, December 26). *Try These Nutrition And Supplement Tips To Keep Your Older Dog Healthy*. PawTracks. https://www.pawtracks.com/dogs/vitamins-for-old-dog/

Cosgrove, N. (2020, December 1). *10 Best Senior Dog Vitamins & Supplements.* Hepper. https://www.hepper.com/best-senior-dog-vitamins-supplements/

Coston, Z. (2022, January 12). *How To Treat Your Dog's Constipation At Home.* Dutch. https://www.dutch.com/blogs/dogs/dog-constipation-home-remedies#

Crow, A., & Winnie. (n.d.). *The Importance Of Exercising Older Dogs.* Senior Tail Waggers. https://seniortailwaggers.com/exercising-older-dogs/

Dog Aging Project. (2020, November 25). *Understanding Behavioral Changes in Senior Dogs.* Dog Aging Project. https://dogagingproject.org/understanding-behavioral-changes-in-senior-dogs/#:~:text=Disorientation%20(staring%20blankly%20at%20walls

Dog Quality. (2020, March 5). *The Do's and Don'ts of Exercising Your Senior Dog.* Dog Quality. https://www.dogquality.co.uk/blogs/news/the-do-s-and-donts-of-exercising-your-senior-dog#:~:text=When%20exercising%20your%20senior%20dog

Donnelly, C., & Evans, J. (2022, December 9). *Discover 7 Natural Remedies to Soothe Your Dog's Itchy Skin.* The Spruce Pets. https://www.thesprucepets.com/home-remedies-for-itchy-dogs-4177184

Driver, K. (2022, December 7). *Is it Time to Say Goodbye? 21 Signs a Dog May Be Dying.* Care Credit. https://www.carecredit.com/well-u/pet-care/signs-a-dog-is-dying/

Farricelli, A. (2022, April 18). *Is My Dog Too Old for a Dental Cleaning?* PetHelpful. https://pethelpful.com/dogs/Is-My-Dog-Too-Old-for-a-Dental-Cleaning

Finlay, K. (2020, May 8). *How to Exercise Your Senior Dog.* American Kennel Club. https://www.akc.org/expert-advice/health/provide-senior-dog-proper-exercise/

Flaim, D. (2016, March 11). *The Importance of Trimming Dog Nails.* Whole Dog Journal. https://www.whole-dog-journal.com/care/nail-clipping/the-importance-of-clipping-dogs-nails/

Flowers, A. (2020, December 1). *Remedies to Relieve Dog Constipation.* Fetch. https://pets.webmd.com/dogs/remedies-dog-constipation

Flowers, A. (2022, November 20). *Hypothyroidism in Dogs.* Fetch. https://pets.webmd.com/dogs/hypothyroidism-in-dogs

Frosek, R. (n.d.). *14 Ways To Improve Your Older Dog's Life.* Modern Dog Magazine. https://moderndogmagazine.com/articles/14-ways-improve-your-older-dogs-life/103806

Gerkensmeyer, R. (2022, December 19). *How to Clean a Dog's Runny Nose.* WagWalking. https://wagwalking.com/grooming/clean-a-dogs-runny-nose

Gerrity, S. (2021, April 27). *How to Create a Pet First Aid Kit, According to a Vet.* Daily Paws. https://www.dailypaws.com/dogs-puppies/health-care/dog-first-aid-emergency/pet-first-aid-kit

Giorgio, K. M. (2021, May 10). *5 Common Senior Dog Health Issues to Watch For.* Daily Paws. https://www.dailypaws.com/dogs-puppies/health-care/senior-dog-health/common-senior-dog-health-issues

Goldstein, L. (2020, December 19). *When to Take Your Dog to the Emergency Vet.* Preventive Vet. https://www.preventivevet.com/dogs/when-to-take-your-dog-to-the-emergency-vet

Grzyb, K. (2018, November 26). *How to Manage Chronic Dog Illnesses Without Getting Overwhelmed.* PetMD. https://www.petmd.com/dog/care/how-manage-chronic-dog-illnesses-without-getting-overwhelmed

Hammers, M. (2017, November 15). *10 Ways to Heal After Losing a Pet.* EverydayHealth. https://www.everydayhealth.com/emotional-health/10-ways-heal-after-losing-pet/

Hartz. (2015, March 13). *How to Treat Your Dog for Intestinal Parasites.* Hartz. https://www.hartz.com/how-to-treat-your-dog-for-intestinal-parasites/#:~:text=Roundworms%20and%20hookworms%20can%20be

Hayes, C. (2020, July 29). *15 things that can make life easier for elderly dogs.* USA Today. https://www.usatoday.com/story/tech/reviewedcom/2020/07/29/15-things-can-make-life-easier-elderly-dogs/5538827002/

Healthy Paws. (n.d.). *Chronic Conditions in Dogs and Cat.* Healthy Paws Pet Insurance. https://www.healthypawspetinsurance.com/chronic-condition-coverage-for-pets#:~:text=Common%20Chronic%20Conditions&text=Diabetes

Heimbuch, J. (n.d.). *7 Things Your Senior Dog Would Like to Tell You.* Old Dog Haven. https://olddoghaven.org/7-things-your-senior-dog-would-like-to-tell-you/

Hitchcock, K. (2020, July 21). *15 Signs Your Dog is Dying: How to Know When Your Dog is Ready to Go.* K9ofmine. https://www.k9ofmine.com/signs-your-dog-is-dying/

The Humane Society Of The United States. (n.d.). *Coping with the death of your pet.* The Humane Society of the United States. https://www.humanesociety.org/resources/coping-death-your-pet

Johnson, M. (2022, March 21). *5 signs of inbreeding in dogs.* PawTracks. https://www.pawtracks.com/dogs/signs-of-inbred-dogs/

Kane, G. (2015, September 25). *Watch for Signs of Health Problems in Older Dogs.* American Kennel Club. https://www.akc.org/expert-advice/health/health-problems-older-dogs-senior-old-age/#:~:text=An%20older%20dog%20is%20more

The Kennel Club. (n.d.). *Inbreeding calculators (COIs)*. The Kennel Club. https://www.thekennelclub.org.uk/health-and-dog-care/health/getting-started-with-health-testing-and-screening/inbreeding-calculators/

Khalsa, D. (2012, November 1). *12 Homeopathic Remedies For Dogs*. Dogs Naturally Magazine. https://www.dogsnaturallymagazine.com/12-homeopathic-remedies/

Klein, J. (2021, October 27). *Dog Euthanasia: When is it Time to Say Goodbye?* American Kennel Club. https://www.akc.org/expert-advice/health/knowing-time-say-goodbye-pet-euthanasia/

Klinger, C. (2018, December 5). *Treating Your Dog's Dry Nose*. Hill's Pet Nutrition. https://www.hillspet.com/dog-care/healthcare/dry-dog-nose-treatments

Kos-Barber, H. (2022, March 2). *Abscesses in Dogs*. PetMD. https://www.petmd.com/dog/conditions/skin/c_dg_abscessation

LakeCross Veterinary. (n.d.). *Signs & How to Treat Bladder Infections in Dogs*. LakeCross Veterinary. https://www.lakecross.com/site/blog-huntersville-vet/2021/09/30/bladder-infection-dog#:~:text=Antibiotics%20are%20the%20number%20one

Lee, C. (2019, January 20). *15 DDR Life Hacks for Deaf Dog Families*. Deaf Dogs Rock. https://deafdogsrock.com/15-ddr-life-hacks-for-deaf-dog-families

Lee, L. (2021, August 17). *Why Is My Dog Coughing, and When Should I Go to the Vet?* GoodRx Health. https://www.goodrx.com/pet-health/dog/dog-coughing

Lin, S. J. (2022, September 27). *My 15-year-old dog has mobility limitations, but these products have dramatically increased his quality of life*. Insider.

https://www.insider.com/guides/pets/senior-dog-mobility-products#a-portable-wagon-with-a-tailgate-3

Marsden, S., Messonnier, S., & Yuill, C. (n.d.). *Veterinary Homeopathy.* VCA Hospitals. https://vcahospitals.com/know-your-pet/veterinary-homeopathy

Mayer, B. (2022, November 9). *Here's what to do if you notice your senior dog coughing and gagging.* PawTracks. https://www.pawtracks.com/dogs/old-dog-coughing-and-gagging/

Meyers, H. (2021, April 6). *Preventing Obesity in Senior Dogs.* American Kennel Club. https://www.akc.org/expert-advice/health/preventing-obesity-in-senior-dogs/

Meyers, H. (2022a, April 26). *Why Do Small Dogs Live Longer Than Large Dogs?* American Kennel Club. https://www.akc.org/expert-advice/health/why-do-small-dogs-live-longer/

Meyers, H. (2022b, August 2). *Why Is My Dog So Itchy? Possible Causes & Treatment.* American Kennel Club. https://www.akc.org/expert-advice/health/why-is-my-dog-so-itchy/

Miller, J. (2016, August 22). *Homeopathic Remedies for Your Dog.* American Kennel Club. https://www.akc.org/expert-advice/health/homeopathic-remedies-for-your-dog/

Nom Nom. (n.d.). *Senior Dog Food Guide for Older Dogs.* Nom Nom Now. https://www.nomnomnow.com/learn/article/senior-dog-food-guide

Oberbauer, A. M., Belanger, J. M., Bellumori, T., Bannasch, D. L., & Famula, T. R. (2015). Ten inherited disorders in purebred dogs by functional breed groupings. *Canine Genetics and Epidemiology, 2*(1). https://doi.org/10.1186/s40575-015-0021-x

Palika, L. (2018, January 12). *7 Ways to Add Joy to Your Old Dog's Life.* The Honest Kitchen. https://www.thehonestkitchen.com/blogs/pet-obsessed/7-ways-to-add-joy-to-your-old-dogs-life

Paul, M. (2015a, June 7). *A Senior Dog Checkup: What to Expect.* Pet Health Network. https://www.pethealthnetwork.com/dog-health/dog-checkups-preventive-care/a-senior-dog-checkup-what-expect

Paul, M. (2015b, August 14). *6 Simple Tips for Exercising Your Senior Dog.* Pet Health Network. https://www.pethealthnetwork.com/dog-health/dog-checkups-preventive-care/6-simple-tips-exercising-your-senior-dog

Pennisi, E. (2017, January 11). *Why large dogs live fast—and die young.* Science. https://www.science.org/content/article/why-large-dogs-live-fast-and-die-young

Pet Basics. (n.d.). *Senior Dog Care: 6 Ways to Promote Healthy Aging.* Pet Basics. https://petbasics.elanco.com/us/health-and-care/senior-dog-care-supplements

Pet Mobility Solutions. (2022, December 27). *5 Things You Must Know Before Buying a Dog Wheelchair.* Handicapped Pets. https://www.handicappedpets.com/blog/5-need-to-know-dog-wheelchair-tips/

Pet Place Veterinarians. (2015, June 8). *14 Common Disorders of Senior Dogs.* Pet Place. https://www.petplace.com/article/dogs/pet-care/14-common-disorders-of-senior-dogs/

Pet Resort. (2017, June 14). *The Most Common Dog Illnesses: Symptoms and Treatment.* Hillrose Pet Resort. https://www.petresort.com/medical/most-common-dog-illnesses-symptoms-treatment/#:~:text=Oral%20infections%20are%20actually%20the

Peters, A. (2022, September 1). *Dog Eye Gunk: What Is It, How to Clean It, and When to Worry.* The Dog People. https://www.rover.com/blog/reviews/dog-eye-gunk/

PetMD Editorial. (2009, March 6). *9 Natural Home Remedies for Your Dog.* PetMD.

https://www.petmd.com/dog/wellness/evr_dg_home_remedi es

PetMD Editorial. (2011, April 26). *Holistic Medicine and How it Can Help Your Pet.* PetMD. https://www.petmd.com/cat/wellness/evr_ct_hollistic_medici ne_and_how_it_can_help_your_pet

Primm, K. (2015, September 30). *From The Vet: 5 Simple Hacks To Make Life Easier For Senior Dogs.* I Heart Dogs. https://iheartdogs.com/simple-life-hacks-to-make-it-easier-for-senior-dogs/

Pulley, K. (2019, March 18). *Home Treatment for a Dog Abscess.* Dogster. https://www.dogster.com/dog-health-care/treat-a-dog-abscess-at-home

Puotinen, C. J. (2017, January 24). *10 Weight Loss Tips for Senior Dogs.* Whole Dog Journal. https://www.whole-dog-journal.com/health/weight_control/10-weight-loss-tips-for-senior-dogs/

Puppy Leaks. (2018, July 5). *10 Tips For Exercising a Senior Dog.* Puppy Leaks. https://www.puppyleaks.com/senior-dog-exercise/

Queen's Park Pet Hospital. (2021, July 20). *Does Your Pet Have an Abscess?* Queen's Park Pet Hospital. https://www.queensparkpethospital.ca/does-your-pet-have-an-abscess/#:~:text=If%20the%20abscess%20hasn

Racine, E. (2019, September 2). *Dog Ear Infections: Symptoms, Causes, Treatment, and Prevention.* American Kennel Club. https://www.akc.org/expert-advice/health/dog-ear-infections/#:~:text=How%20are%20Dog%20Ear%20Infectio ns

Randall, S. (2022, June 6). *10 Essential Home Remedies for Dogs to Have at Home.* Top Dog Tips. https://topdogtips.com/home-remedies-for-dogs/

Reisen, J. (2022, October 4). *Physical and Mental Signs that Your Dog is Aging.* American Kennel Club. https://www.akc.org/expert-advice/health/physical-mental-signs-dog-aging/

Robinson, L., Segal, J., & Segal, R. (2019). *Coping with Losing a Pet.* Help Guide. https://www.helpguide.org/articles/grief/coping-with-losing-a-pet.htm

Royal Veterinary College. (n.d.). *Dry eye in dogs.* Royal Veterinary College. https://www.rvc.ac.uk/small-animal-vet/teaching-and-research/fact-files/keratoconjuncitivitis-sicca-dry-eye#:~:text=Dry%20eye%20is%20usually%20treated

Rubin, J. L. (n.d.). *If Your Pet Is Officially Part Of The Senior Community, You Should Check Out These 21 Products.* BuzzFeed. https://www.buzzfeed.com/julialynnrubin/helpful-products-for-senior-pets

Simon, L. (2021, October 28). *Natural Cough Remedies in Dogs - Conditions Treated, Procedure, Efficacy, Recovery, Cost, Considerations, Prevention.* Wag Walking. https://wagwalking.com/treatment/natural-cough-remedies

Small Door Veterinary. (n.d.-a). *Exercise Needs for Puppies, Adults and Senior Dogs.* Small Door Veterinary. https://www.smalldoorvet.com/learning-center/wellness/exercise-needs-dog-lifestages

Small Door Veterinary. (n.d.-b). *Senior Dogs 101: What changes can I expect in my senior dog?* Small Door Veterinary. https://www.smalldoorvet.com/learning-center/dogs/changes-to-expect-senior-dog

Small Door Veterinary. (n.d.-c). *Senior Dogs 101: Tips to keep your senior dog healthy as they age.* Small Door Veterinary. https://www.smalldoorvet.com/learning-center/seniors/keep-senior-dog-healthy

Smith, A. (2023, January 1). *25 Best Senior Dog Supplements in 2023.* Discover Magazine.

https://www.discovermagazine.com/lifestyle/25-best-senior-dog-supplements-in-2022

Stuart, A. (2010, March 17). *How to Figure Out Your Dog's Age.* WebMD. https://pets.webmd.com/dogs/how-to-calculate-your-dogs-age

Tasaki, S. (2022, December 28). *Mental Stimulation for Senior Dogs: Tips to Keep Older Dogs Busy.* The Wildest. https://www.thewildest.com/dog-lifestyle/mental-stimulation-for-senior-dogs

Tracey, A., & Valentini, K. (2022, February 9). *How to Recognize & Treat a Dog UTI.* Daily Paws. https://www.dailypaws.com/dogs-puppies/health-care/dog-conditions/dog-uti

Turner, B. (2021, July 17). *Your Dog Has Diarrhea: What to Do and NOT Do.* Preventive Vet. https://www.preventivevet.com/dogs/your-dog-has-diarrhea-what-to-do

Turner, B. (2022, September 20). *Bad Breath... It's NOT Always Their Teeth.* Preventive Vet. https://www.preventivevet.com/dogs/bad-breath-not-always-teeth

Vecchioni, H. (n.d.). *How to Groom a Dog's Nose.* Daily Puppy. https://dogcare.dailypuppy.com/groom-dogs-nose-3879.html

Ventiera, S. (2021, June 1). *Products and Techniques to Support Your Older Dog.* AARP. https://www.aarp.org/home-family/friends-family/info-2021/products-for-older-dogs.html

Veterinaire Pet Care. (n.d.). *Vet Services for Acute Illnesses.* Veterinaire Pet Care. https://veterinairepetcare.com/acute-illnesses-management.html

Wag! (n.d.). *How to Shave a Small Dog's Face.* WagWalking. https://wagwalking.com/grooming/shave-a-small-dogs-face#:~:text=Hold%20his%20head%20still%20and

Weir, M., & Panning, A. (n.d.). *Instructions for Ear Cleaning in Dogs.* VCA Animal Hospitals. https://vcahospitals.com/know-your-pet/instructions-for-ear-cleaning-in-dogs

Williams, K., & Downing, R. (n.d.). *Feeding Mature and Senior Dogs.* VCA Animal Hospitals. https://vcahospitals.com/know-your-pet/feeding-mature-and-senior-dogs

Williams, K., & Downing, R. (2009). *Obesity in Dogs.* VCA Animal Hospitals. https://vcahospitals.com/know-your-pet/obesity-in-dogs

Williams, K., & Ward, E. (2009). *Hypothyroidism in Dogs.* VCA Animal Hospitals. https://vcahospitals.com/know-your-pet/hypothyroidism-in-dogs

Wilson, W. B. (2019, November 15). *Senior Dog Food: What Is the Best Thing to Feed an Old Dog?* BeChewy. https://be.chewy.com/best-senior-dog-food-choosing-the-best-dog-food-for-older-dogs/

Winter Park Veterinary Hospital. (n.d.). *Canine Chronic Disease Management.* Winter Park Veterinary Hospital. https://wpvet.com/general-care/chronic-disease-management/canine-chronic-disease-management/

Image References

Bigandt_Photography. (2015). *Old Staffordshire Bull Terrier* [Image]. iStock. https://www.istockphoto.com/photo/senior-staffordshire-bull-terrier-gm494571264-77521367?phrase=old%20dog

freestocks. (2020). *Dog with Intravenous Line* [Image]. Pexels. https://www.pexels.com/photo/dog-with-intravenous-line-on-his-leg-4074725/

Glinskaia, E. (2021). *Grooming* [Image]. iStock. https://www.istockphoto.com/photo/animal-groomer-shaved-dog-with-electric-shaver-machine-in-cabinet-at-vet-clinic-gm1317747825-405085360

Liukov. (2020). *Disabled Dog* [Image]. iStock. https://www.istockphoto.com/photo/the-dog-is-disabled-the-dog-is-in-a-wheelchair-gm1282821930-380437623

Richards, A. (2017). *Boston Terrier In Car* [Image]. Unsplash. https://unsplash.com/photos/aYHgchNOsGY

RossHelen. (2021). *Dog Having Teeth Brushed* [Image]. iStock. https://www.istockphoto.com/photo/dog-ready-for-teeth-brushing-gm1324673256-409931328

Simpson, J. (2020). *Walking Dog on Lead* [Image]. Unsplash. https://unsplash.com/photos/8MGPoUWuePA

Wandler, M. (2022). *Dog Collar with Red Rose* [Image]. iStock. https://www.istockphoto.com/photo/dog-collar-with-a-red-rose-symbolizing-love-gm1420593110-466522775

Ward, E. (2018). *Retriever Hug* [Image]. Unsplash. https://unsplash.com/photos/ISg37AI2A-s

Zontica. (2020). *Dog Paws with Healthy Food* [Image]. iStock. https://www.istockphoto.com/photo/healthy-natural-pet-food-in-bowl-and-dogs-paws-on-yellow-background-gm1284996229-381967478?phrase=dog%20healthy